Cataract Management in Demanding Cases - Pediatric and Refractive Cataract Surgery

Edited by Canan Aslı Utine Yıldırım and Melis Palamar Onay

Published in London, United Kingdom

Cataract Management in Demanding Cases - Pediatric and Refractive Cataract Surgery
http://dx.doi.org/10.5772/intechopen.1009048
Edited by Canan Aslı Utine Yıldırım and Melis Palamar Onay

Contributors
Adel Ebraheem, Amr Saad, Arañó Ferrer Jerónimo, Ata Baytaroğlu, Detlev R. H. Breyer, Shimin Wu, Xiaoqin Yan

First published in London, United Kingdom, 2026 by IntechOpen
IntechOpen is the global imprint of INTECHOPEN LIMITED, registered in England and Wales, registration number: 11086078, 167-169 Great Portland Street, London, W1W 5PF, United Kingdom

For EU product safety concerns: IN TECH d.o.o., Prolaz Marije Krucifikse Kozulić 3, 51000 Rijeka, Croatia, info@intechopen.com or visit our website at intechopen.com.

British Library Cataloguing-in-Publication Data
A catalogue record for this book is available from the British Library

Cataract Management in Demanding Cases - Pediatric and Refractive Cataract Surgery
Edited by Canan Aslı Utine Yıldırım and Melis Palamar Onay
p. cm.
Print ISBN 978-1-83634-974-7
Online ISBN 978-1-83634-973-0
eBook (PDF) ISBN 978-1-83634-975-4

Meet the editors

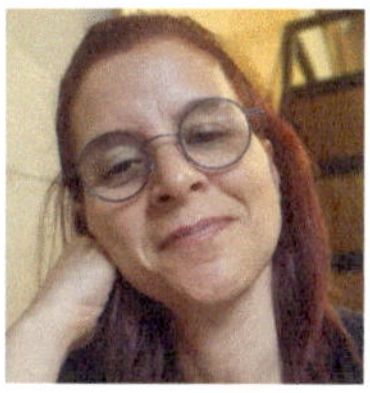

Dr. Utine Yıldırım has expertise in cataract, glaucoma, and corneal transplantation, with more than 20,000 surgical cases. She performs high-risk surgeries that need a multi-disciplinary approach. She has vast experience in premium (multifocal) lens implantation for refractive cataract surgery, as well as in kerato-refractive surgery, including femto-LASIK, SMILE, and PRK; transscleral sutured intraocular lens implantation; internal fixation of subluxated or dislocated lenses; aniridia-correcting IOL implantation; and pediatric cataract surgery. Her primary expertise lies in the field of medical and surgical treatment of corneal pathologies. She holds a Master's degree in Biomedical Engineering. Currently, her h-index is 27, and her i10-index is 45. She has 2376 citations.

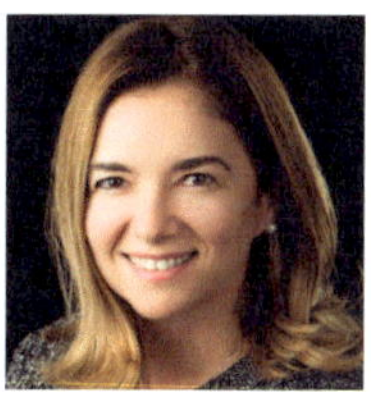

Melis Palamar Onay, Prof, MD, is the Secretary of the Turkish Ophthalmology Association, Cornea and Ocular Surface Division. She is an expert on Cornea and Ocular Surface, Ocular Oncology, and Ocular Infections. She has 177 articles on PubMed. Her h-index is 25, and her i10-index is 62. She has 2389 citations. She is the owner and the Assistant Editor of the journals *European Eye Research and European Transplant Research*.

Contents

Preface

Cataract surgery has long been regarded as a simple procedure with excellent results. This understanding creates a massive demand and a hidden burden for surgeons. However, in some cases, such as pediatric eyes, there are inherent challenges, including differences in corneal and ocular biomechanics, incomplete development, and time constraints due to the risk of amblyopia. Furthermore, recent advancements in lens technology have paved the way to refractive excellence in far, intermediate, and near distances. This paradigm shift in cataract surgery necessitates considering additional details.

This book covers important topics about the management of cataract in pediatric eyes and in patients with high refractive demands. These include preoperative evaluation, surgical tips and techniques, and postoperative care. We believe this book will help cataract surgeons refine and polish their approaches to these complex cases, where small tips and tricks can change clinical outcomes.

We cordially thank Ms. Marica Novakovic for her tireless and dedicated help during the editorial process.

Dr. Canan Aslı Utine Yıldırım, MD, MSc
Professor,
Faculty of Medicine,
Department of Ophthalmology,
İzmir Biomedicine and Research Center,
Dokuz Eylül University,
İzmir, Türkiye

Dr. Melis Palamar Onay, MD
Professor,
Faculty of Medicine,
Department of Ophthalmology,
Ege University,
İzmir, Türkiye

Section 1

Pediatric Cataract Surgery – Main Principles and Challenges

Chapter 1

Preoperative Evaluation of Pediatric Cataracts

Ata Baytaroğlu

Abstract

Pediatric cataracts, whether congenital or juvenile, constitute a leading cause of preventable visual loss and therefore pose serious challenges to families, clinicians, and public health systems. Early identification of pediatric cataracts and timely intervention are essential, as any delay may result in permanent vision loss and hinder a child's development. Due to the anatomy and physiology of a child's growing eye, proper preoperative evaluation is crucial for a successful surgical outcome. Preoperative evaluation of pediatric cataracts involves a thorough history and clinical examination, precise biometry for IOL planning, differential diagnosis, and active parental involvement. Challenges include managing developmental factors and postoperative complications. Technological advances have improved surgical outcomes, and early intervention is crucial for preventing amblyopia and enhancing visual and cognitive functions. The central questions of this chapter are: What are the differences in preoperative evaluation in adult and pediatric cataract cases? When and to what extent is systemic evaluation necessary? How should IOL selection and timing be after the surgical decision? What can be evaluated preoperatively to reduce postoperative complications?

Keywords: congenital, juvenile, cataracts, IOL calculation, preoperative examination

1. Introduction

The clinical management of pediatric cataracts involves several components, including skills, facilities, patient access to care, and postoperative compliance. There are varying causes and prevalences in different regions, making preoperative examination protocols even more critical. Successful surgical management and postoperative rehabilitation of pediatric cataracts depend upon the accuracy of preoperative evaluation. Visual acuity outcomes are significantly affected by age at the time of diagnosis, and improved visual acuity outcomes have been correlated with increased improvements in pediatric intraocular lens technology and small incision cataract surgeries. Although techniques such as capsulorhexis have yielded improved visual outcomes and a decrease in complication rates, posterior capsular opacification (PCO) and subsequent secondary surgery continue to be a leading concern, leading to the implementation of primary posterior capsulectomy in younger cataract patients. While better outcomes have been found in children with earlier diagnosis of pediatric cataracts who are under the age of two, optimal protocols and treatments remain a

IntechOpen

matter of considerable debate, leaving room for future investigations in both unilateral versus bilateral cases and a more precise comparison of primary and secondary implantation techniques in pediatric cataract surgery.

2. Definition and classification of pediatric cataracts

A comprehensive definition for pediatric cataracts clarifies the two different types, congenital and juvenile, which differ in terms of clinical significance. Congenital cataracts are present at birth, and juvenile cataracts begin postnatally. This differentiation is significant because, depending on the timing of presentation, the management will differ, and the patient's vision can range from normal to the need for aggressive management. Congenital cataracts will need immediate treatment to prevent long-term visual deprivation amblyopia, and juvenile cataracts are treated more at the physician's discretion because they present more variably [1].

Centrally located cataracts with >3 mm diameter opacities are indisputably surgical, whereas peripheral, small, and partial cataracts often do not require surgery because their visual outcome is more favorable. In this chapter, the evaluation of such cases that do not require surgery but require close follow-up will not be discussed [2, 3].

Further clarification must also be provided concerning congenital versus juvenile cataracts for treatment protocol differences due to the unique presentations of congenital cataracts. When cataracts are present with microphthalmia or persistent fetal vasculature, this occurs predominantly in congenital cataracts. These cases need comprehensive evaluation, and a multidisciplinary approach with ophthalmology and other related specialists must be implemented. This approach necessitates genetic counseling and systemic evaluation, as these factors can greatly impact postoperative surgical results [4, 5].

Pediatric cataracts are also variable regarding laterality, with about 64.3% of patients having bilateral cataracts versus 35.7% with unilateral cataracts [1, 6]. Unilateral cataracts require more aggressive postoperative visual rehabilitation to ensure proper visual development. The most common morphological classification of pediatric cataracts is zonular, at 33.8%. However, there are varying morphologies, such as nuclear, polar, lamellar, and total (**Figure 1**). The morphologies have extremely variable natural histories and difficulties regarding surgery and postoperative care [4, 6–9]. An example would be a total cataract that obstructs visual stimuli from reaching the neural tissue of the eye. Immediate removal of these dense cataracts will need to be performed to preserve vision because the cataract acts as a dark barrier against visual development. Polar cataracts have some potential for visual rehabilitation while maintaining some vision due to their location (inferior polar) compared to superior polar. The location determines what kind of effects will be shown, but it should also be noted that morphological classification also helps discern between causes. For example, bilateral, symmetrical cataracts can signify genetic or systemic metabolic diseases. On the other hand, unilateral, dense cataracts presented at an early age might be from infectious and developmental causes [1].

The most significant cause of pediatric cataracts is idiopathic, at 72.5%, which means that no cause has been found upon diagnosis. Genetic and systemic causes account for 19% of secondary pediatric cataract causes. In underdeveloped countries where vaccination and health services are limited, infectious diseases may be the cause of an infantile cataract [1, 10].

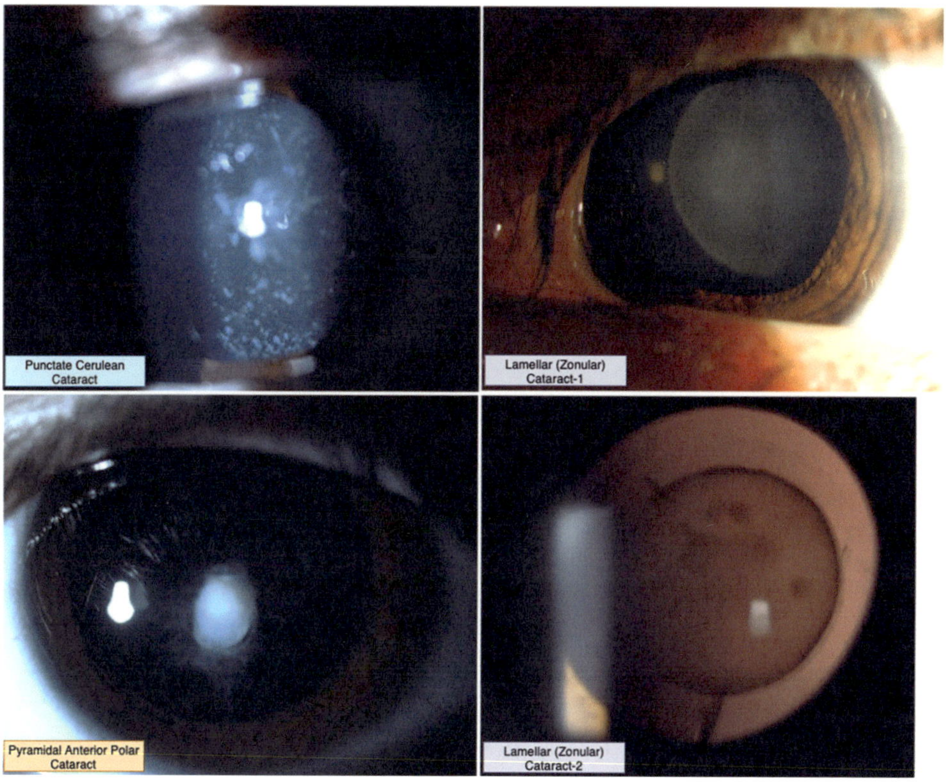

Figure 1.
Most common pediatric cataract types.

There are many associations with pediatric cataracts. Other conditions, such as strabismus (52.2%) and nystagmus (24.37%), can be identified in conjunction. Most often, strabismus and nystagmus indicate prolonged amblyopia and visual deprivation in children due to a disruption of their visual pathway neurogenesis [11–14]. In a follow-up of about 20 years, manifest nystagmus occurred in about 1/3 of the bilateral congenital cases, regardless of the timing of surgery, and surgery performed at less than 2 months of age did not prevent it. In addition, the presence of preoperative nystagmus is not necessarily a risk factor for poorer visual acuity outcome [13].

Numerous systemic conditions and congenital syndromes are also associated with pediatric cataracts. Therefore, the inclusion of both ocular and extraocular manifestations in classification and definition can help anticipate surgical complications and postoperative difficulties with visual rehabilitation. All children with pediatric cataracts should undergo a general medical workup to rule out these associations and prevent life-threatening complications.

The estimated global prevalence ranges from 1 to 15 cases per 10,000 children, with 200,000 children globally being blind secondary to bilateral cataract. These are not actual global rates due to reporting and variance in risk factors and populations in certain areas [7, 8, 15]. Globally, this underscores the need for screening and appropriate referral pathways for prompt care. Childhood cataract is the most frequent cause of treatable childhood blindness and is therefore considered a public health concern. The incidence of childhood cataract and its contribution to childhood blindness are much greater in developing countries than in the developed world, where lack of education, late presentation, lack of specialists, and barriers to access all have an influence. In Asia alone, the prevalence of childhood blindness has surpassed the one million cases mark, and cataract accounts for a substantial percentage of this, with India, for example, contributing about 7.4–15.3% [9]. The mean age of presentation is 6 years. However, preterm children are four times more likely to develop bilateral congenital or infantile cataract if born before 33 weeks [16]. The risk of congenital and infantile cataract is also greater for children whose mothers experience pregnancy complications. Up to 67% of mothers of children with congenital cataract have had illnesses in pregnancy, and 22% have taken medicines in pregnancy. 22% of congenital cataracts have an associated systemic abnormality, and 27% are associated with ocular abnormalities [9]. Therefore, prenatal diagnosis is vital in detecting prenatal abnormalities that may increase the risk of cataract formation.

Detailed preoperative evaluation is also practical in predicting certain postoperative complications, making the preoperative evaluation the most critical period for ensuring maximum neurodevelopmental outcomes and adequate visual skills. Among the common postoperative complications, rates for postoperative posterior capsular opacification (PCO) in the pediatric population range from 21 to 51.1% [6, 12, 17]. Secondary glaucoma is not an uncommon outcome in children needing earlier surgery and, similar to PCO, this is dependent upon several factors such as etiology, age, type of cataract, etc.

3. Clinical assessment and planning

The preoperative evaluation of pediatric cataracts significantly differs from that of adults due to several unique anatomical, physiological, and developmental considerations. Since the first thing that comes to mind when we talk about cataract surgery is senile cataract in adults and elderly patients, we prefer to mention the clinical evaluation in pediatric cases, especially the important points that distinguish them from adults. A brief summary of these fundamental differences is listed in the **Table 1**.

Aspect	Pediatric cataracts	Adult cataracts
anatomy	Smaller, less rigid structures, a more elastic lens capsule	Larger and more rigid lens and ocular structures
Inflammatory response	More pronounced, higher risk of complications	Less pronounced
Systemic evaluation	Frequently required to exclude related cases	Rarely needed
IOL calculation	More complex due to ongoing eye growth	Usually standard
Timing	Urgent to prevent amblyopia	Rarely urgent
Surgical technique	Necessity for additional procedures like anterior vitrectomy, posterior capsulorhexis	Mostly standard
IOL implantation	Age-dependent, often delayed in infants	Mostly simultaneous
Post-op	Intensive, long-term follow-up, amblyopia management	Routine follow-up

Table 1.
Key differences between pediatric and adult cataracts.

Feature	Adult cataract	Pediatric cataract
Lens material	Typically hard and dense. Requires phacoemulsification to break up.	Often soft and "gummy." Requires irrigation-aspiration or vitrectomy for removal.
Lens size	Average diameter ~ 9.3 mm at 16 years.	Average diameter ~ 6.0–7.0 mm at birth, rapidly growing in the first 2 years.
Lens capsule	Thicker and less elastic.	Thinner and more elastic, making capsulorhexis more challenging due to the tendency for "runaway" tears.
Scleral rigidity	Higher, more rigid.	Lower, more elastic, and less rigid, leading to a greater tendency for collapse during surgery and higher vitreous pressure.
Corneal rigidity	Higher.	Lower, less likely to self-seal after incisions.
Anterior chamber	More stable.	Often unstable due to low scleral rigidity and increased vitreous upthrust.
Iris	Less vascular, generally less reactive post-surgery.	Thicker and more vascular, leading to a higher incidence of postoperative inflammation.
Axial length of globe	Stable (average ~ 23–24 mm).	Rapidly growing (17–17.5 mm at birth, increasing significantly in early years), impacting IOL power calculation.
Posterior capsule opacification (PCO)	Common, but usually managed with Nd:YAG laser capsulotomy.	Much higher incidence and often more aggressive due to increased cellular proliferation; frequently requires surgical intervention at the time of initial cataract surgery.
Associated ocular anomalies	Less common, unless related to trauma or systemic disease.	More frequently associated with other ocular abnormalities like microcornea, aniridia, coloboma, and persistent fetal vasculature (PFV).
Visual pathway development	Fully developed.	Still developing, highly susceptible to amblyopia if vision is deprived by the cataract. This necessitates prompt surgical intervention for visually significant cataracts.
Postoperative inflammation	Present, but generally more predictable.	Increased tissue reactivity often leads to more significant fibrinous or exudative postoperative uveitis.

Table 2.
Differences in adult and pediatric cataracts.

Type of cataract	Associated causes	Notes
Anterior polar cataract (**Figure 1**)	• Genetics: Often autosomal dominant inheritance, sporadic cases also exist.	• Usually small and localized. • May be associated with other anterior segment abnormalities. • Often visually insignificant, but monitor for progression.
Posterior polar cataract	• Genetics: Autosomal dominant inheritance is common, but sporadic forms occur. Genes like PITX3, MAREF, and members of the CRY (crystallin) gene family are implicated. • May also be associated with persistent fetal vasculature (PFV), posterior lenticonus/lentiglobus, aniridia, Lowe syndrome, Rothmund-Thomson syndrome.	• Central, discoid opacity at the posterior pole. • High risk of posterior capsular rupture during surgery due to strong adherence to the capsule. • Can cause significant visual impairment, even if small, due to its central location.

Type of cataract	Associated causes	Notes
Nuclear cataract	• Genetic: Mutations in crystallin genes (CRYAA, CRYAB, CRYBB1, CRYBB2, CRYGC, CRYGD, CRYGS) are common. • Metabolic: Galactosemia (classic "oil droplet" cataract), Lowe syndrome (oculocerebrorenal syndrome). • Infections: Congenital rubella syndrome (can also be lamellar or total). • Syndromes: Down syndrome.	• Opacity, primarily affecting the central nucleus of the lens. • Can be present at birth or develop later. • Varies in density and visual impact.
Lamellar (Zonular) Cataract (**Figure 1**)	• Genetic: Most common form of hereditary cataract, frequently autosomal dominant. Mutations in crystallin genes are often involved. • Metabolic: Hypoglycemia, hypocalcemia, galactosemia (can be lamellar in later stages). • Infections: Congenital rubella syndrome.	• Opacity in one or more concentric layers (lamellae) of the lens, typically sparing the very center (nucleus) and the outermost cortex. • Often bilateral and progressive. • Visual significance depends on the density and extent of the opacity.
Cortical cataract	• Trauma: Blunt or penetrating ocular trauma. • Metabolic: Diabetes (often bilateral, "snowflake" cataracts), hypocalcemia. • Inflammation: Chronic uveitis (e.g., juvenile idiopathic arthritis-associated uveitis). • Medications: Steroid use (especially prolonged systemic or topical use). • Radiation exposure.	• Opacities in the lens cortex, often appearing as spokes or wedges radiating inward. • Can progress to involve the entire lens.
Posterior subcapsular cataract (PSC)	• Steroid use: Most common acquired cause in children. • Trauma: Blunt ocular trauma. • Inflammation: Chronic uveitis (especially JIA-associated). • Metabolic: Diabetes. • Genetic: Some genetic syndromes (e.g., Alport syndrome, Fabry disease).	• Opacity located directly beneath the posterior capsule, often granular or vacuolated. • Can cause significant glare and reduced vision, especially in bright light or with near vision. • Tends to progress rapidly.
Total/Complete cataract	• Severe forms of other types: Any of the above types can progress to a total cataract if left untreated or if the underlying cause is severe. • Congenital Rubella Syndrome: Often causes dense, white total cataracts. • Persistent fetal vasculature (PFV): Unilateral, dense white cataract with associated retrolental fibrovascular membrane. • Severe metabolic disorders: Untreated galactosemia. • Genetic syndromes: Many severe genetic syndromes can lead to total cataracts.	• The entire lens is opaque, appearing white or milky. • Causes profound visual deprivation and amblyopia if not treated promptly.

Type of cataract	Associated causes	Notes
Membranous cataract	• Trauma: Often follows significant trauma that causes lens capsule rupture and subsequent absorption of lens material, leaving a thick fibrous membrane. • Inflammation: Severe, chronic intraocular inflammation. • Post-surgical: Can form after inadequate removal of lens material or complications. • Congenital: Less common, may result from severe intrauterine insult or complete liquefaction and absorption of lens material.	• A thin, fibrous membrane replaces the normal lens, often with minimal or no remaining lens cortex/nucleus. • Can be visually significant and challenging to manage surgically.
Punctate cataract (**Figure 1**)	• Genetic: Often inherited, sometimes associated with chromosomal abnormalities or syndromes (e.g., Down syndrome, Nance-Horan syndrome). • Metabolic: Hypocalcemia, Fabry disease.	• Small, discrete, dot-like opacities scattered throughout the lens. • Usually visually insignificant unless numerous and dense. •
Coronary cataract	• Genetic: Often inherited, typically not associated with systemic disease.	• Club-shaped opacities arranged radially in the deep cortex, surrounding the nucleus. • Usually develops later in childhood or adolescence. Often visually insignificant.
Sutural cataract	• Genetic: Often inherited.	• Opacities involving the Y-sutures of the lens. • Typically visually insignificant.

Table 3.
Morphological types of cataracts and their systemic associations.

3.1 Anatomy

The crystalline lens is a transparent, biconvex structure that can develop opacities that vary in morphology, including total, zonular (such as lamellar), and capsular cataracts (including both anterior and posterior subcapsular types). Morphological variations impact not only the optical quality of the lens but also surgical approaches when removal or intraocular lens (IOL) implantation is necessary [1]. Thus, for ease of understanding, we have presented the differences from adult cataract and the systemic or genetic conditions that may be associated with different cataract morphologies in **Tables 2** and **3**.

3.2 Inflammatory response

To understand the inflammatory response in pediatric cataracts, it is essential to consider both the causes and the management of inflammation post-surgery. Pediatric cataract surgery often results in a heightened inflammatory response due to the immature anatomical structures in children and the presence of other ocular abnormalities [18]. This inflammation can lead to several complications, including posterior capsule opacification (PCO), visual axis opacification, and secondary glaucoma. The intensity of postoperative inflammation has been documented to be particularly severe in children, occurring in about 13.8% of operated eyes, a figure that increases to approximately 15.9% when anterior vitrectomy is performed [19].

Several factors exacerbate the inflammatory response following surgery. The presence of ocular trauma, commonly seen in pediatric traumatic cataracts, can significantly complicate the inflammatory landscape due to damage to corneal and uveal structures. Such cases often present with elevated inflammatory markers, increasing the difficulty of surgical interventions [20]. The surgical approach itself influences inflammation levels; for example, techniques involving intracameral injection of medications like triamcinolone acetonide have been shown to reduce postoperative inflammation effectively. Intracameral corticosteroids can lead to "quiet eyes" with minimized signs of inflammation post-surgery, suggesting their integral role in managing postoperative care [21]. Moreover, the presence of coexisting conditions, such as uveitis, can heighten the risk of developing cataracts and complicate the management of inflammatory responses. Chronic inflammatory conditions like juvenile idiopathic arthritis (JIA) can make cataract surgery more complex and increase the risk of postoperative complications [22, 23].

We believe it is essential to reiterate the importance of both preoperative and postoperative inflammation control in uveitic patients. In these cases, it is necessary to ensure that adequate immunosuppressive treatment is initiated prior to surgery using a multidisciplinary approach. Inflammation control has a dramatic impact on surgical technique, IOL selection, and implantation decisions, as well as postoperative complications in these cases. Current research recommends against the utilization of an intraocular lens (IOL) in patients exhibiting active uveitis despite optimal pharmacological intervention, very young children, hypotonic eyes, rubeotic eyes, those with uveitis of indeterminate etiology, and instances where IOL-associated complications have arisen in the contralateral eye. The data recommend less invasive small incision cataract surgery with foldable intraocular lens, particularly in unilateral cataract cases, provided that the uveitis is appropriately managed and the patient is systemically stable [22].

3.3 Systemic evaluation

Although systemic evaluation is crucial in pediatric cataract cases, underlying causes can be found in 60% of bilateral cases and 50% of unilateral cases, even in the most successful series [24]. Congenital cataract and persistent fetal vasculature (PFV) generally manifest within the first year of life and necessitate prompt surgical intervention. The age at which idiopathic and hereditary cataracts are presented varies significantly, and the time of surgery is contingent upon the visual significance of the cataract.

A pivotal aspect of managing pediatric cataracts lies in understanding their genetic underpinnings. Research has demonstrated that pediatric cataracts exhibit considerable phenotypic and genetic heterogeneity, with numerous loci identified as contributing to this disorder. Unfortunately, our current knowledge is limited, especially regarding multisystem triggers, as data on systemic associations with pediatric cataracts is still insufficient [25, 26]. Genetically, pediatric cataracts have been linked to a range of inherited conditions. Research indicates that approximately 10 to 29% of pediatric cataracts have identifiable genetic causes, with over 200 syndromes associated with their development [25, 27].

Metabolic causes represent another significant component in the multifactorial etiology of pediatric cataracts. Conditions like type 1 diabetes mellitus have been shown to precipitate cataracts in pediatric patients, occurring either at the onset of diabetes or within years following diagnosis [28]. Furthermore, metabolic disorders such as galactosemia and hereditary hyperferritinemia-cataract syndrome highlight how metabolic dysregulation can lead to cataract formation through oxidative stress and lens protein aggregation [12, 24, 25]. A comprehensive metabolic screening is thus recommended for children presenting with bilateral cataracts to rule out associated metabolic conditions. Infections encountered during pregnancy or early in a child's life, such as those caused by the rubella virus, have also been established as notable risk factors for developing pediatric cataracts [1]. Finally, acquired causes, particularly traumatic incidents, contribute significantly to the pediatric cataract population. Trauma accounts for approximately 30% of pediatric cataracts, making it a considerable factor in childhood visual impairment [29]. The recommended evaluation for bilateral cataracts in the absence of a family history comprises a urine analysis for reducing sugars, TORCH screening (toxoplasmosis, rubella, cytomegalovirus, varicella), a Venereal Disease Research Laboratory (VDRL) test for syphilis, and a blood assay for calcium, phosphorus, glucose, and galactokinase levels. Further comprehensive evaluation should be conducted in collaboration with the pediatrician and geneticist.

In summary, pediatric cataracts result from a complex interaction of genetic, metabolic, infectious, and traumatic factors. A systematic evaluation that includes genetic testing, metabolic profiling, and comprehensive clinical assessments remains crucial for developing effective treatment strategies and improving visual outcomes in affected children. However, for practical guidance, we have not included the differential diagnosis of over 100 defined syndromes here, as 60% of bilateral cataracts and 80% of unilateral cases are diagnosed as idiopathic.

3.4 Mimicking conditions

The differential diagnosis of pediatric cataracts includes a wide range of conditions such as idiopathic causes, genetic factors, maternal infections, metabolic disorders, trauma, and systemic diseases. Many diseases can also mimic cataracts. A key feature of these conditions is leukocoria. The laterality of the lesion is crucial when considering differential diagnoses. Among pediatric cases, retinoblastoma is the most critical disease to identify, as it can imitate and cause cataracts. Differentiating retinoblastoma is vital because it is a life-threatening condition that requires prompt treatment. Additionally, retinoblastoma may present with secondary glaucoma, uveitis, and other ocular issues, which could be mistaken for cataracts [30, 31].

Retinopathy of prematurity (ROP) is an important differential diagnosis for cataracts in patients with a history of premature birth, low gestational weight, and developmental delay. This is because, in most cases, by the time it appears similar to cataracts, it is accompanied by retinal detachment at stages 4–5 and indicates a poor prognosis. ROP and other retinal lesions may be linked to cataract formation, especially after surgeries like vitrectomy. Studies show that about 19% of patients who have had lens-sparing vitrectomy for ROP develop cataracts [32].

Persistent fetal vasculature (PFV) is another condition that can present with leukocoria and is also a common pseudoretinoblastoma. PFV is more frequently seen in children under 1 year old and typically presents unilaterally in full-term infants without systemic associations. In children aged 2–5 years, Coats' disease becomes a more common cause of leukocoria and retinal detachment, often mimicking the appearance of cataracts. Coats' disease is also exclusively unilateral and occurs more often in males. Again, in this age group, familial exudative vitreoretinopathy (FEVR), a developmental retinal vascular anomaly, can be seen as an ocular media opacity resembling cataracts, along with retinal detachment in stages 3 and more advanced stages. In children older than 5 years, ocular toxocariasis should also be considered. It can cause a cataract-like appearance due to vitreous inflammation and retinal lesions [31, 33]. Less commonly, posterior lenticonus and iris melanocytomas can also be considered among the lesions that cause cataracts or a cataract-like appearance [34, 35].

Consequently, accurate diagnosis requires a combination of clinical examination and the use of multimodal imaging techniques to differentiate these conditions and ensure appropriate management. Ocular ultrasonography, computed tomography, or MRI, and anterior segment optical coherence tomography are essential and critical for distinguishing these conditions from cataracts.

3.5 IOL calculation

Intraocular lens (IOL) calculation in pediatric cataract surgery presents unique challenges due to the ongoing growth and refractive changes in children's eyes. Children's eyes are still growing, which affects the accuracy of IOL power calculations. This necessitates age-appropriate adjustments and undercorrection strategies to account for future myopic shifts. In pediatric cataract surgery, performing calculations without planning the patient's age and future emmetropic status may result in serious amblyopia [36, 37]. Pediatric eyes pose unique challenges due to their smaller size, changing axial length, and corneal curvature. Accurate measurements of axial length and keratometry are crucial for precise IOL power calculation. Although much more challenging to perform, immersion techniques are more accurate than contact applanation techniques for measuring axial length [38].

At this point, the most critical decision for selecting the right IOL is to use the correct formulation. In a study comparing 16 methods, including both traditional and novel formulations, the Hoffer Q formula was found to be the most successful in terms of achieving predicted values. In contrast, the SRK/T formulation was the furthest from the expected target. However, it is essential to emphasize that the difference between these two extremes is an average of 0.21 diopters, and no data on long-term outcomes have been presented [39, 40]. A recent systematic review also reported successful results with Barrett Universal II (BUII), Hoffer Q, and SRK/T formulations, emphasizing that the best postoperative values were obtained with BUII [40]. Moreover, a meta-analysis reported the top three formulas to be BUII, SRK/T, and Holladay 1, in respective order [41].

We have summarized the comparison of these four formulas recommended in the studies in the **Table 4**.

The key points in IOL selection can be broken down into two crucial aspects:

Undercorrection strategy: A common approach involves undercorrecting the IOL power to allow for the natural growth of the eye, reducing the risk of myopic shifts. However, age at surgery significantly influences the refractive outcomes. Children below 2 years of age tend to experience more hypermetropia post-surgery, whereas in children ≤1 year old, a larger myopic shift, with the mean myopic shift being −6.4 diopters, has been reported [42]. There is no significant difference in the myopic shift or postoperative visual acuity between children who received full correction and those who were undercorrected by 2 diopters or more. This suggests that undercorrection does not adversely affect visual outcomes compared to full correction [43].

Formula	Strengths	Limitations
Hoffer Q	High accuracy in shorter axial lengths, good overall performance	Variability in very young children
SRK/T	Reliable for older children and longer axial lengths	Undercorrection tendency in younger children
Barrett Universal II	High predictive accuracy, suitable for a wide range of axial lengths	Requires careful biometry for best results
Holladay 1	Good performance in average axial lengths	Less effective in very short or very long eyes

Table 4.
IOL calculation formula comparison.

The generally recommended undercorrection method is to aim for 20% undercorrection in children under 2 years of age and 10% undercorrection in children between 2 and 8 years of age, or to achieve a postoperative refraction equivalent of 7 minus the current years of age. As a common point among all these formulations, it can be said that it is reasonable to aim for undercorrection of 1–4 diopters, depending on the surgeon's patient-based preference [44–46].

Formula selection: No single formula is perfect for all pediatric cases. The choice often depends on the child's age, axial length, and specific ocular parameters. Newer formulas like Barrett Universal II and Kane show promise, but traditional formulas like Hoffer Q and SRK/T remain widely used due to their proven track records.

3.6 IOL choice and timing

The standard of care in congenital cataracts, undisputedly, is to operate on unilateral cataracts by 6 weeks old and bilateral cataracts by 10 weeks old. For bilateral aphakia, secondary IOL implantation between the ages of 2 and 6 years can achieve comparable visual outcomes. Early surgery (before 30 days of age) and lack of primary IOL implantation are associated with a higher risk of postoperative glaucoma, and primary IOL implantation can reduce this risk [47–49].

Timing for IOL implantation in pediatric cataracts is a contentious topic among ophthalmic specialists. Current trends increasingly favor primary IOL implantation during cataract extraction, particularly for children over 6 months old, as they have been associated with better visual outcomes compared to secondary implantation [50, 51]. A longitudinal study involving a Swedish pediatric cataract registry demonstrated that 71.6% of children underwent primary IOL implantation [51]. However, there remain concerns regarding potential complications associated with primary IOL implantation, particularly in very young patients. For instance, some studies have shown a higher rate of reoperations in infants under 7 months old who received primary IOLs [52]. Thus, decisions must consider individual patient factors, such as ocular health, systemic conditions, and the potential for inflammation, especially in cases with uveitis [53]. In contrast, secondary IOL implantation can reduce the risk of complications, including secondary glaucoma, particularly in complex cases. A retrospective analysis indicated that while there is a general trend toward primary IOL implantation, many pediatric patients remain aphakic for extended periods, with only 24% receiving a secondary IOL within 5 years after lensectomy due to parental preferences or anticipated lack of benefit [54]. The planning of cataract surgery and IOL implantation in pediatric cataract cases is summarized as a flowchart in **Figure 2**.

The choice of IOL type is equally significant in pediatric cataract management, with factors such as material compatibility, risk of posterior capsule opacification (PCO), and economic considerations playing vital roles. Hydrophobic acrylic IOLs are

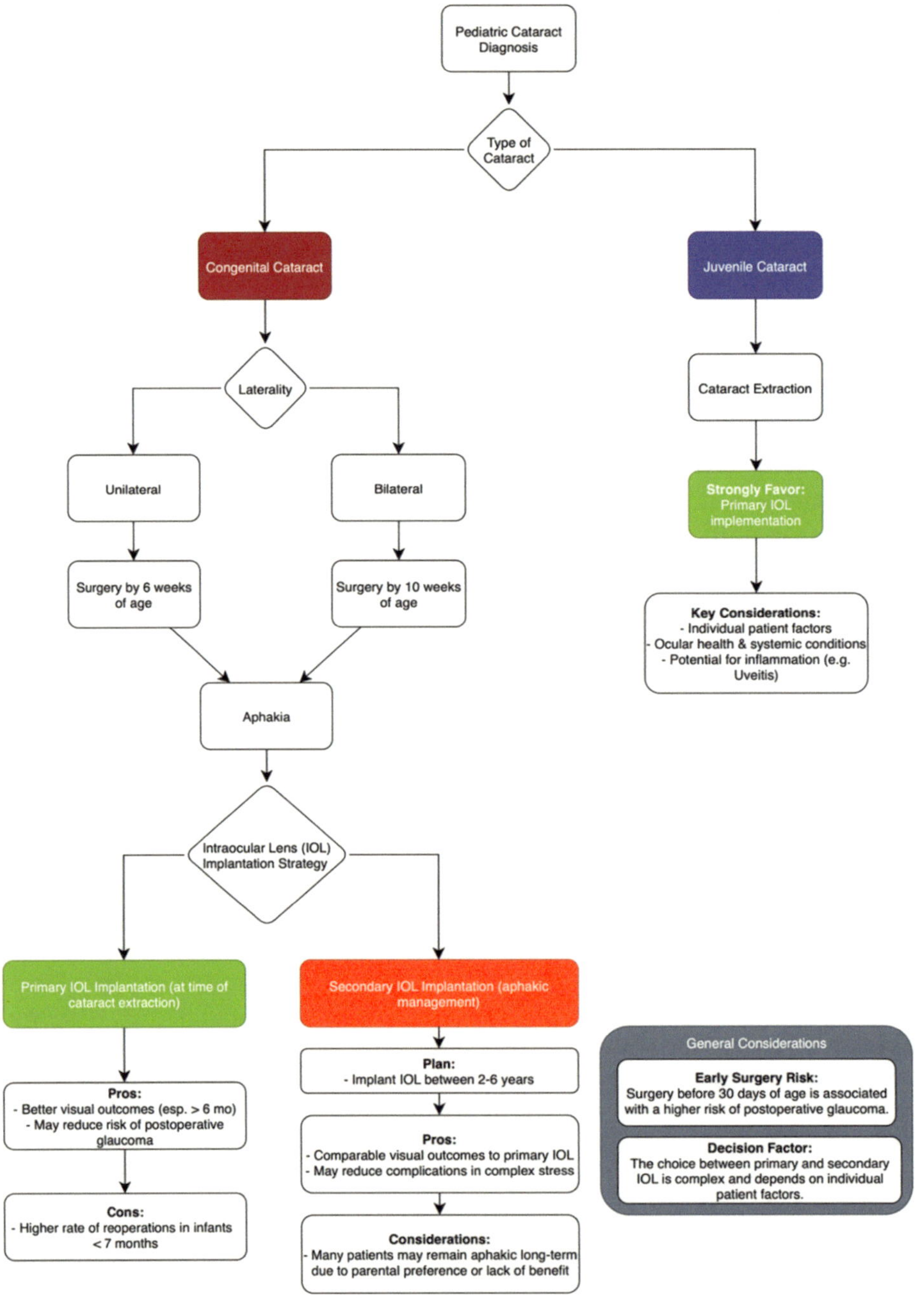

Figure 2.
Basic flow chart for approaching pediatric cataract cases.

often favored for their lower rates of PCO compared to hydrophilic lenses. Studies have indicated that hydrophobic IOLs, particularly those with specific edge designs, outperform their hydrophilic counterparts in preventing PCO, making them a preferable choice in many pediatric cases [55]. Additionally, the implantation technique is pivotal. Primary in-the-bag implantation remains the gold standard (**Figure 3**), particularly when sufficient capsular support is maintained. However, the use of sulcus fixation has been shown to reduce risks in cases where capsular integrity is compromised [56].

Another current and controversial topic is multifocal IOL implantation in pediatric cataract cases. It is a complex and evolving area of ophthalmology. These premium IOLs aim to provide multiple focal points, potentially improving both near and distance vision. Studies have shown significant improvements in visual acuity post-implantation. For instance, one study reported that 79% of eyes with bilateral cataracts achieved a best-corrected distance visual acuity of 20/40 or better, and 26% achieved 20/20 [57]. Another study found that 90.91% of patients showed significant improvement in visual acuity in all three (distance-intermediate-near) distances [58]. Improvement in stereopsis and binocularity was also reported in these studies [57–59]. Although multifocal IOL implantation appears to solve many different problems at once, it remains an uncharted zone due to the lack of long-term results and the unknown effects of orthoptic treatment, which is often required, especially in unilateral cases.

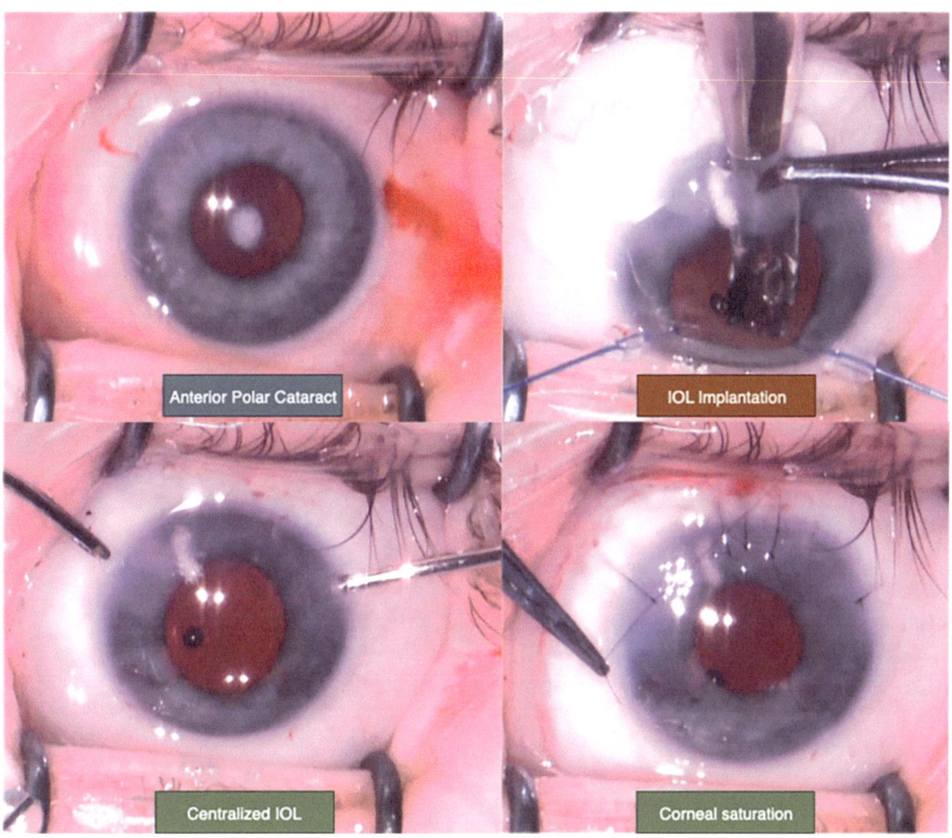

Figure 3.
Anterior polar cataract extraction and simultaneous IOL implantation.

Understanding the visual anatomy and requirements of the individual child influences the decision-making process around IOL types based on age-related factors and anticipated long-term outcomes. In summary, IOL implantation timing and choice in pediatric cataracts must be tailored to the child's individual clinical scenario while weighing the benefits of early correction against potential complications.

4. Conclusion

A comprehensive history and careful clinical examination are essential to address questions regarding the cause of the cataract, whether to operate, when to operate, and how to operate. Preoperative biometry is crucial for determining the specifics of the intraocular lens implant and the postoperative target refraction. Pediatric cataracts can be associated with various systemic conditions, including genetic syndromes, metabolic disorders, and infections. Early diagnosis and prompt surgical intervention are critical to prevent irreversible amblyopia. The timing of surgery should be carefully considered based on the onset, duration, and morphology of the cataract. Preoperative imaging with tools like OCT can provide valuable information about the lens and capsule, reducing intraoperative risks and surprises. Genetic testing is recommended for unexplained bilateral cataracts, while metabolic and infectious testing should be guided by clinical context. In summary, successful management of pediatric cataracts relies on thorough preoperative evaluation, careful planning, and individualized care. Collaboration with pediatricians and genetic counselors, along with advancements in imaging and surgical techniques, can significantly improve outcomes for children with cataracts.

Author details

Ata Baytaroğlu
Department of Ophthalmology, Hacettepe University, Ankara, Turkey

*Address all correspondence to: abaytaroglu@hacettepe.edu.tr

References

[1] Tartarella MB, Britez-Colombi GF, Milhomem S, Lopes MCE, Fortes Filho JB. Pediatric cataracts: Clinical aspects, frequency of strabismus and chronological, etiological, and morphological features. Arquivos Brasileiros de Oftalmologia. 2014;**77**(3):143-147

[2] Birch EE, Subramanian V, Patel CC, Stager D. Preoperative visual acuity and contrast sensitivity in children with small, partial, or non-central cataracts. Journal of American Association for Pediatric Ophthalmology and Strabismus. 2013;**17**(4):357-362

[3] Choi J, Kim JH, Kim SJ, Yu YS. Clinical characteristics, course, and visual prognosis of partial cataracts that seem to be visually insignificant in children. Journal of American Association for Pediatric Ophthalmology and Strabismus. 2012;**16**(2):161-167

[4] Chen J, Lin H, Chen W. Perioperative challenges and solutions in the management of children with cataracts. Pediatric Lens Diseases. 2016:121-127

[5] Berdahl JP, Vann RR. Cataract surgery: Preoperative evaluation. In: Essentials of Cataract Surgery. Boca Raton: CRC Press; 2024. pp. 9-24. Available from: https://www.taylorfrancis.com/books/9781003524038/chapters/10.1201/9781003524038-2

[6] Chattannavar G, Badakere A, Mohamed A, Kekunnaya R. Visual outcomes and complications in infantile cataract surgery: A real - world scenario. BMJ Open Ophthalmology. 2022;7(1):e000744

[7] Medsinge A, Nischal KK. Pediatric cataract: Challenges and future directions. Clinical Ophthalmology. 2015;**9**:77-90

[8] Trivedi RH, Wilson ME. Pediatric Cataract: Preoperative Issues and Considerations. Pediatric Ophthalmology: Current Thought and A Practical Guide; 2009. pp. 311-324

[9] Katre D, Selukar K. The prevalence of cataract in children. Cureus. 2022

[10] Poschkamp B, Dinkulu S, Böckermann C, Mukwanseke E, Paschke C, Hopkins A, et al. Management of Bilateral Congenital and Juvenile Cataracts in a low-income country: Patient identification, treatment outcomes, and follow up. Children. 2024;**11**(9):1064

[11] Villanueva MJR, Santiago APD. Effects of prolonged waiting time on visual outcomes of patients with pediatric cataract in a tertiary public hospital. Acta Medica Philippina. 2024;**58**(16):77-84. Available from: https://actamedicaphilippina.upm.edu.ph/index.php/acta/article/view/8653

[12] Moreira J, Ribeiro I, Mota Á, Gonçalves R, Coelho P, Maio T, et al. Cataratas em Idade Pediátrica: Estudo Retrospetivo de 12 Anos (2004-2016). Acta Médica Portuguesa. 2017;**30**(3):169-174

[13] Young MP, Heidary G, VanderVeen DK. Relationship between the timing of cataract surgery and development of nystagmus in patients with bilateral infantile cataracts. Journal of American Association for Pediatric Ophthalmology and Strabismus. 2012;**16**(6):554-557

[14] Kemmanu V, Khanum A, Madhavrao B, Raghunandan N, Muthu S, Venkatesh R, et al. Outcome of pediatric cataract surgery including color vision, stereopsis, and cognition in a tertiary eye care center in India. Oman Journal of Ophthalmology. 2024;**17**(2):237-244

[15] Bhayana A, Dhull C, Khokhar SK. Preoperative evaluation and investigative modalities in pediatric cataract. Essentials of Pediatric Cataract Surgery. 2021:3-20

[16] Al-Damri A, Alotaibi HM. Congenital cataracts in preterm infants: A review. Cureus. 2023;**15**(6):e40378

[17] Aldamri A, AlKhaldi SA, AlQahtani DS, AlShaalan KS, Alshamrani M. Long-term outcome and determinants of primary pediatric cataract surgery. Saudi Journal of Ophthalmology. 2024;**38**(3):252-256

[18] Gasper C, Trivedi RH, Wilson ME. Complications of pediatric cataract surgery. Developments in Ophthalmology. 2016;**57**:69-84

[19] Chia WA, Martin F. Childhood cataracts. Clinical & Experimental Ophthalmology. 2001;**29**(2):75-80

[20] Günaydın NT, Oral AYA. Pediatric traumatic cataracts: 10-year experience of a tertiary referral center. BMC Ophthalmology. 2022;**22**(1):199

[21] Mohamed TA, Soliman W, Fathalla AM. Effect of intracameral triamcinolone acetonide on postoperative intraocular inflammation in pediatric traumatic cataract. European Journal of Ophthalmology. 2016;**26**(2):114-117

[22] Phatak S, Lowder C, Pavesio C. Controversies in intraocular lens implantation in pediatric uveitis. Journal of Ophthalmic Inflammation and Infection. 2016;**6**(1):12

[23] Bajraktari G, Jukić T, Kalauz M, Oroz M, Bertetić AR, Vukojević N. Evaluation of postoperative outcomes after cataract surgery in patients with juvenile idiopathic arthritis-associated uveitis. European Journal of Ophthalmology. 2025;**35**(3):1109-1116

[24] Nihalani BR, VanderVeen DK. Systemic and ocular associations in pediatric patients undergoing cataract surgery. Graefe's Archive for Clinical and Experimental Ophthalmology. 2023;**261**(1):241-246

[25] Tan Y, Hu LY, Shen YY, Chen H, Zou YS, Luo LX, et al. Hotspots and frontiers of genetic research on pediatric cataracts from 2013 to 2022: A scientometric analysis. International Journal of Ophthalmology. 2023;**16**(10):1682-1691

[26] Zin OA, Neves LM, Motta FL, Horovitz DDG, Guida L, Gomes LHF, et al. Novel mutation in CRYBB3 causing pediatric cataract and microphthalmia. Genes (Basel). 2021;**12**(7):1069

[27] Neves LM, Pinto M, Zin OA, Cunha DP, Agonigi BNS, Motta FL, et al. The cost of genetic diagnosis of suspected hereditary pediatric cataracts with whole-exome sequencing from a middle-income country perspective: A mixed costing analysis. Journal of Community Genetics. 2024;**15**(3):235-247

[28] Wilson ME, Levin AV, Trivedi RH, Kruger SJ, Elliott LA, Ainsworth JR, et al. Cataract associated with type-1 diabetes mellitus in the pediatric population. Journal of American Association for Pediatric Ophthalmology and Strabismus. 2007;**11**(2):162-165

[29] Ambroz SC, Töteberg-Harms M, Hanson JVM, Funk J, Barthelmes D, Gerth-Kahlert C. Outcome of pediatric cataract surgeries in a tertiary center in Switzerland. Journal of Ophthalmology. 2018;**2018**:1-10

[30] Mirzayev I, Gündüz AK, Biçer Ö, Tarlan B. The final diagnosis: Retinoblastoma or pseudoretinoblastoma. Journal of Pediatric Ophthalmology and Strabismus. 2021;**58**(3):161-167

[31] Shields CL, Schoenberg E, Kocher K, Shukla SY, Kaliki S, Shields JA. Lesions simulating retinoblastoma (pseudoretinoblastoma) in 604 cases. Ophthalmology. 2013;**120**(2):311-316

[32] Ezisi CN, Kekunnaya R, Jalali S, Balakrishnan D, Kumari PR, Mohamed A, et al. Cataract surgery in children with retinopathy of prematurity (ROP): Surgical outcomes. British Journal of Ophthalmology. 2017;**101**(8):1128-1131

[33] Vinekar A, Wu WC, Lorenz B, Bavaskar S, Berrocal A, Lopez-Cañizares A, et al. Rare pediatric retinal diseases: A review. Indian Journal of Ophthalmology. 2025;**73**(5):622-636

[34] Agarwal R, Jain V, Kaur M, Titiyal JS. Atypical presentation of peripheral posterior lenticonus and role of multi-modal ocular imaging in its diagnosis and management. BML Case Reports. 2021;**14**(2):e238801

[35] Al-Kharashi A, Alsakran WA, Alshamrani AA, AlZaid A, Maktabi AMY, Alzahrani YA. Iris melanocytoma in a child: Clinical and histopathological findings. American Journal of Case Reports. 2021;**22**:e931385

[36] Touzé R, Dureau P, Edelson C, Borella Y, Barjol A, de Laage de Meux P, et al. Congenital cataract surgery: Long-term refractive outcomes of a new intraocular lens power correction formula. Acta Ophthalmologica. 2022;**100**(8):e1641-e1645

[37] Kaur S, Sukhija J, Ram J. Intraocular lens power calculation formula in congenital cataracts: Are we using the correct formula for pediatric eyes? Indian Journal of Ophthalmology. 2021;**69**(12):3442-3445

[38] Heede S, Astle WF, Hackenberg L, Ruddell S, Kim A. The comparative accuracy of four IOL power calculation formulas in pediatric eyes undergoing cataract surgery. Clinical and Surgical Ophthalmology. 2011;**29**(10-11):220-227

[39] Achiron A, Yahalomi T, Biran A, Levinger E, Cohen E, Elbaz U, et al. A comprehensive evaluation of 16 old and new intraocular lens power calculation formulas in pediatric eyes. Clinical Ophthalmology. 2024;**18**:2225-2238

[40] Stopyra W, Grzybowski A. Intraocular lens power calculation formulas in children—A systematic review. Journal of Clinical Medicine. 2024;**13**(15):4400

[41] Hong Y, Sun Y, Xiao B, Ainiwaer M, Ji Y. A Bayesian network meta-analysis on comparisons of intraocular lens power calculation methods for paediatric cataract eyes. Eye. 2023;**37**(16):3313-3321

[42] Panahibazaz M, Mohammadpour S, Samaeili A. Overcoming myopic shift by the initial inductive hypermetropia in pediatric cataract surgery. Indian Journal of Ophthalmology. 2021;**69**(12):3515-3519

[43] Lambert SR, Archer SM, Wilson ME, Trivedi RH, del Monte MA, Lynn M. Long-term outcomes of undercorrection versus full correction after unilateral intraocular lens implantation in children. American Journal of Ophthalmology. 2012;**153**(4):602-608.e1

[44] Enyedi LB, Peterseim MW, Freedman SF, Buckley EG. Refractive changes after pediatric intraocular lens implantation. American Journal of Ophthalmology. 1998;**126**(6):772-781

[45] VanderVeen DK. Predictability of intraocular lens calculation and early refractive status. Archives of Ophthalmology. 2012;**130**(3):293

[46] Sachdeva V, Katukuri S, Kekunnaya R, Fernandes M, Ali MH. Validation of guidelines for undercorrection of intraocular lens power in children. American Journal of Ophthalmology. 2017;**174**:17-22

[47] Hu K, Zhang Y, Chen W, Chen H, Wang Q, He A, et al. Visual acuity and complications at age 7 years following bilateral secondary intraocular lens implantation at 2 to younger than 6 years for Pediatric Aphakia. JAMA Ophthalmology. 2025;**143**(7):570-576

[48] Lin D, Liu Z, Chen J, Lin Z, Zhu Y, Chen C, et al. Practical pattern of surgical timing of childhood cataract in China: A cross-sectional database study. International Journal of Surgery. 2019;**62**:56-61

[49] Mataftsi A, Haidich AB, Kokkali S, Rabiah PK, Birch E, Stager DR, et al. Postoperative glaucoma following infantile cataract surgery. JAMA Ophthalmology. 2014;**132**(9):1059

[50] Zhao QH. Commentary review: Challenges of intraocular lens implantation for congenital cataract infants. International Journal of Ophthalmology. 2021;**14**(6):923-930

[51] Yen KG, Repka MX, Sutherland DR, Haider KM, Hatt SR, Kraker RT, et al. Complications occurring through 5 years following primary intraocular lens implantation for pediatric cataract. JAMA Ophthalmology. 2023;**141**(8):705

[52] Magnusson G, Haargaard B, Basit S, Lundvall A, Nyström A, Rosensvärd A, et al. The paediatric cataract register (PECARE): An overview of operated childhood cataract in Sweden and Denmark. Acta Ophthalmologica. 2018;**96**(1):51-55

[53] Terrada C, Julian K, Cassoux N, Prieur AM, Debre M, Quartier P, et al. Cataract surgery with primary intraocular lens implantation in children with uveitis: Long-term outcomes. Journal of Cataract and Refractive Surgery. 2011;**37**(11):1977-1983

[54] Repka MX, Dean TW, Kraker RT, Li Z, Yen KG, de Alba Campomanes AG, et al. Visual acuity and ophthalmic outcomes 5 years after cataract surgery among children younger than 13 years. JAMA Ophthalmology. 2022;**140**(3):269

[55] Zhao Y, Yang K, Li J, Huang Y, Zhu S. Comparison of hydrophobic and hydrophilic intraocular lens in preventing posterior capsule opacification after cataract surgery. Medicine. 2017;**96**(44):e8301

[56] Liu Z, Lin H, Jin G, Tan X, Qu B, Jin L, et al. In-the-bag versus ciliary sulcus secondary intraocular lens implantation for pediatric aphakia: A prospective comparative study. American Journal of Ophthalmology. 2022;**236**:183-192

[57] Huang Y, Dong X, Zhang J, Wan X, Wang M, Xie L. Full-diffractive multifocal intraocular lens posterior optic capture for selected pediatric cataracts. Journal of Refractive Surgery. 2021;**37**(6):390-397

[58] Jiang M, Zhang J, Ding Y, Huang Y. Multifocal intraocular lens implantation in children with unilateral congenital cataracts. Journal of Cataract and Refractive Surgery. 2024;**50**(1):18-23

[59] Du Q, Ding Y, Liu X, Huang Y. Comparison of the axial growth with multifocal and monofocal intraocular lenses in unilateral pediatric cataract surgery. Graefe's Archive for Clinical and Experimental Ophthalmology. 2024;**262**(12):3889-3896

Chapter 2

Pediatric Cataract in Type 1 Diabetes Mellitus: Clinical Challenges and Surgical

Shimin Wu and Xiaoqin Yan

Abstract

This chapter systematically examines the distinct pathophysiological mechanisms underlying cataract development in children with Type 1 Diabetes Mellitus (T1DM), while establishing evidence-based protocols for preoperative evaluation and optimized perioperative glycemic management. Special focus is given to surgical challenges unique to diabetic pediatric populations, including compromised corneal endothelial cell density and heightened risks of vitreous liquefaction, with comparative analysis of biocompatibility profiles for various intraocular lens materials. Clinically validated approaches are presented regarding: (1) Adjusted phacoemulsification parameters for diabetic lenses (2) Modified primary posterior continuous curvilinear capsulorhexis (PCCC) techniques (3) Targeted postoperative anti-inflammatory regimens The chapter culminates in proposing a multidisciplinary collaborative framework (endocrinology, ophthalmology, pediatric) for personalized postoperative surveillance, emphasizing dynamic monitoring of diabetic retinopathy progression and refractive status evolution.

Keywords: pediatric, type 1 diabetes mellitus (T1DM), cataract, cataract surgery, long-term management

1. Introduction

Cataracts in pediatric patients with type 1 diabetes mellitus (T1DM) can be categorized into early and late onset [1]. Early-onset cataracts in children with T1DM represent a particularly rare complication, especially when they manifest within the initial 6 months following the onset of diabetes [2, 3]. The incidence of this condition is influenced by a multitude of factors, including age, gender, geographic region, and race, yet comprehensive data remain unavailable [4–6]. Various studies have examined the prevalence and incidence of pediatric cataracts in T1DM, utilizing data from extensive pediatric cohorts and registries. The prevalence of early diabetic cataracts in this population ranges from 0.7 to 3.4% among children and adolescents with T1DM [3]. In contrast, late-onset cataracts are recognized as a long-term complication, typically emerging a decade after the initial diabetes diagnosis, akin to patterns observed in adult diabetes [7].

The pathophysiological mechanisms underlying early diabetic cataracts remain incompletely elucidated [2]. Nonetheless, several hypotheses have been proposed regarding their etiology, including osmotic damage, the polyol pathway, and oxidative stress [8–10]. The development of cataracts in children with T1DM continues to be an area of active investigation. Hyperglycemia, a hallmark of diabetes, plays a significant role in the pathogenesis of diabetic cataracts. During hyperglycemia, the altered metabolism of excess glucose leads to localized disruptions to fiber cell morphology and cell swelling in the outer cortex of the lens. This damage is thought to result from

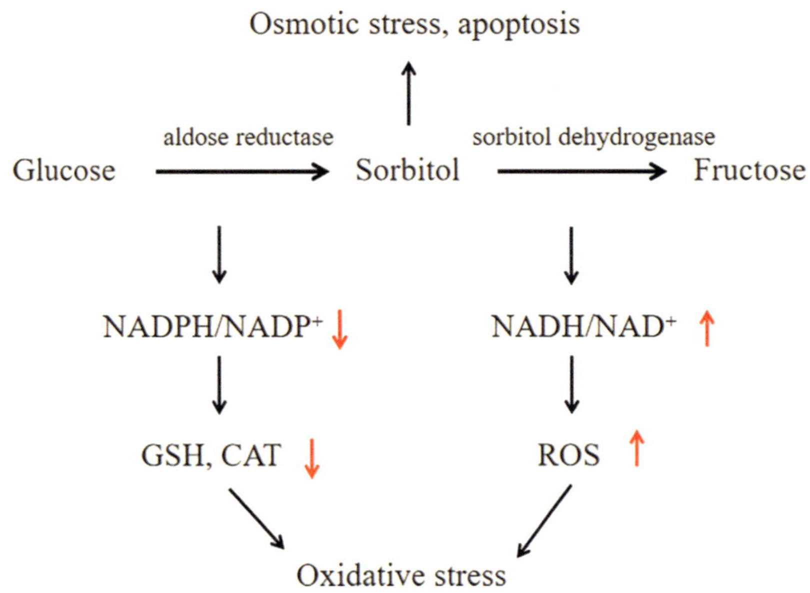

Figure 1.
Schematic diagram of polyol pathway and oxidative stress [11].

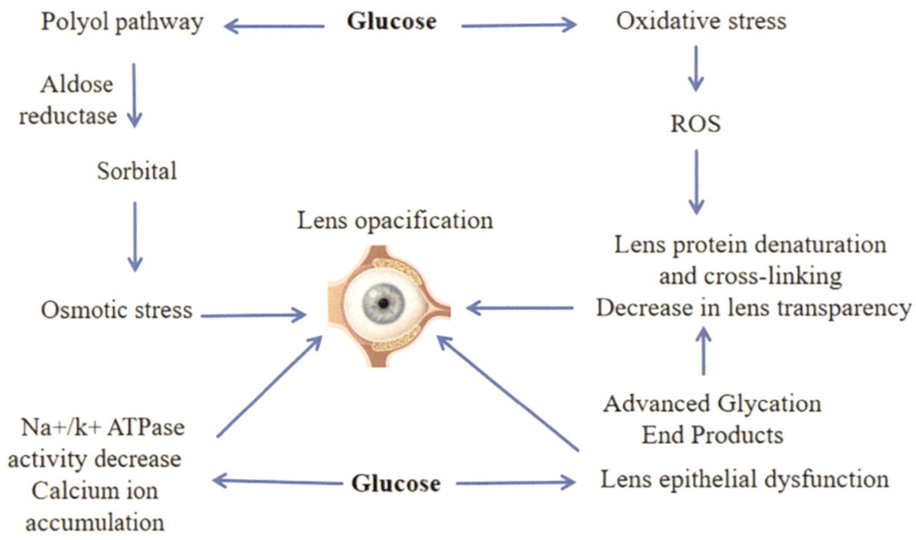

Figure 2.
Schematic diagram of the pathogenesis of diabetic cataract.

osmotic stress and oxidative stress due to the accumulation of intracellular sorbitol, the depletion of NADPH, and the generation of fructose metabolites *via* the polyol pathway (**Figures 1** and **2**) [11–13]. In children with type 1 diabetes, the rate of cataract development shows a peak at diabetes onset and declines with longer diabetes duration. This suggests that hyperglycemia-induced osmotic damage to lens fibers at the onset of diabetes might be the main pathomechanism [3].

2. Clinical manifestations

In pediatric patients with T1DM, cataracts can be categorized into early-onset and late-onset types. The development of diabetic cataracts in this population often serves as an initial indicator of T1DM or manifests within 6 months following the diagnosis. The primary clinical manifestations include diminished visual acuity and alterations in the lens structure. Typically, early-onset cataracts are bilateral and characterized by snow-flake-like opacities in the posterior subcapsular region. These cataracts are generally diagnosed concurrently with T1DM or within the first 6 months post-diagnosis. Their rapid and frequently irreversible progression, which persists despite optimal glycemic management through contemporary insulin therapies, implies that lens fiber damage may occur due to undetected hyperglycemia prior to the formal diagnosis of diabetes. Additionally, some patients experience cataracts that can advance and mature swiftly, occasionally within days, particularly during adolescence. A preceding event may include the abrupt onset of myopia, attributed to alterations in the lens's optical density. In examining the morphology of early diabetic cataracts, various forms have been identified, including posterior subcapsular, lamellar, cortical, snowflake, and milky white types. However, most other researchers recognize fewer types, with posterior subcapsular cataracts being the most frequently reported form in pediatric diabetic patients.

Clinical and individual characteristics indicate that female gender, adolescence, a prolonged history of hyperglycemic symptoms, and elevated HbA1c levels at the time of diabetes diagnosis are significant risk factors for cataract development. Conversely, the incidence of ketoacidosis at diabetes onset appears to be lower in these patients [3]. The youngest patients documented in the literature with early diabetic cataracts are as young as 5 years old, although the majority are adolescents [14–16]. Iafusco et al. noted an equal gender distribution in the pediatric population with type 1 diabetes mellitus (T1DM) and early diabetic cataracts, whereas other studies have reported a predominance of female patients [14, 16, 17]. This group of authors also observed the occurrence of ketoacidosis as an indicator of decompensated T1DM in all patients, aligning with the findings of most earlier studies [16]. Recent studies have intriguingly indicated a reduced incidence of ketoacidosis [9, 18]. Additionally, there exists considerable variability in hemoglobin A1c (HbA1c) levels both at the time of diabetes diagnosis and at the onset of early diabetic cataracts [2, 15].

Late cataracts, akin to diabetic cataracts observed in adults, represent a long-term complication, sharing similar clinical manifestations and typically emerging approximately 10 years following the diagnosis of type 1 diabetes [7].

3. Differential diagnosis

Cataracts in children can arise from various causes, including type 1 diabetes, which is associated with endocrine and metabolic disorders such as hypocalcemia, hypoglycemia, and other conditions like atopic dermatitis and corticosteroid use [19].

3.1 Metabolic disorders

Metabolic disorders are significant contributors to cataract formation, particularly those affecting carbohydrate, amino acid, calcium, and copper metabolism. In infants, galactosemia, specifically galactose-1-phosphate uridyl transferase deficiency, is a critical consideration. This condition typically results in zonular cataracts, characterized by haziness or opacification of the perinuclear lens layers and sometimes the nucleus. Early-stage cataracts may exhibit an oil droplet appearance, detectable with a fully dilated pupil, and can progress to complete lens opacification within weeks. However, early intervention with a galactose-free diet can potentially reverse these lens changes. In cases of galactokinase deficiency, cataracts represent the primary clinical manifestation. These cataracts are typically zonular and can manifest within the first few months or years of life, or later during childhood.

Neonatal hypoglycemia is also linked to the early onset of cataracts, and ketotic hypoglycemia has been associated with cataract formation as well. There is a well-established association between cataracts and hypocalcemia. Patients with hypoparathyroidism may exhibit various types of lens opacities.

The oculocerebral renal syndrome of Lowe is characterized by the presence of cataracts in infants, with affected male children often presenting with dense bilateral cataracts at birth, frequently accompanied by glaucoma and miotic pupils. Heterozygous females commonly exhibit punctate lens opacities.

The characteristic sunflower cataract associated with Wilson disease is infrequently observed in children. Additionally, various lens opacities can occur in children with certain sphingolipidoses, mucopolysaccharidoses, and mucolipidoses, particularly in conditions such as Niemann-Pick disease, mucosulfatidosis, Fabry disease, and aspartylglycosaminuria.

3.2 Drugs, toxic agents, and trauma

Among the various pharmacological and toxic agents capable of inducing cataracts, corticosteroids hold significant importance within the pediatric population. Steroid-induced cataracts are typically characterized by posterior subcapsular lens opacities, with variability in both incidence and severity. The relative contributions of factors such as dosage, mode of administration, treatment duration, and individual susceptibility remain subjects of debate, and the pathogenesis of steroid-induced cataracts has yet to be fully elucidated. The impact on visual acuity is contingent upon the extent and density of the lens opacity, with many cases resulting in only minimal to moderate impairment. Notably, there is potential for reversibility in some instances of steroid-induced cataracts. It is imperative that children undergoing prolonged steroid therapy undergo regular ophthalmic evaluations.

Ocular trauma is another significant etiological factor for cataracts in children, with lens opacification potentially arising from either blunt or penetrating injuries. Furthermore, cataracts may serve as a critical indicator of child abuse.

Cataract formation following exposure to therapeutic radiation is contingent upon both the dose and duration of exposure, with adult studies indicating a 50% incidence rate at a lens dose of 15 Gy. A delayed onset is typically observed in these cases.

4. Treatment

Surgical intervention for cataracts in pediatric patients with T1DM requires a meticulous and individualized approach. Early surgical intervention is essential to prevent amblyopia and optimize visual outcomes. Compared to the general population, diabetic patients face increased risks associated with cataract surgery [20]. Therefore, it is critical for ophthalmologists to conduct a comprehensive preoperative assessment, taking into account the timing and selection of intraocular lenses, as well as addressing any pre-existing diabetic ocular conditions. Intraoperatively, particular attention must be paid to achieving adequate pupillary dilation and considering the potential need for adjunctive surgical procedures [20]. Postoperative care should involve vigilant monitoring for complications such as pseudophakic cystoid macular edema, diabetic macular edema, and posterior capsular opacification. Surgical techniques and postoperative management strategies are continually evolving, integrating both conventional practices and innovative advancements derived from adult cataract surgery. Currently, there is no unified set of indications for surgical treatment. For further details, please consult "the Chinese Expert Consensus on the Perioperative Management of Cataracts in Children (2022)", "Update on pediatric cataract surgery", and so on. [21–23].

For children unable to cooperate with vision tests, dense nuclear cataracts are present, characterized by turbidity along the visual axis with a diameter exceeding 3 mm. This lens opacity impedes both fundus and refractive examinations and is often associated with strabismus, amblyopia, and nystagmus, resulting in an inability to maintain a fixed gaze. In contrast, children who can cooperate with vision tests exhibit a best corrected visual acuity of less than 0.4 due to lens abnormalities for those with type 1 diabetic cataracts, elective surgical intervention is advised once blood sugar levels are stably controlled.

Cataract surgery is generally conducted *via* small, self-sealing corneal incisions, thereby obviating the necessity for sutures. Contemporary cataract surgery employs phacoemulsification, a technique that utilizes ultrasonic waves delivered through a handheld probe to disintegrate the opacified lens into smaller fragments *via* a circular anterior capsulotomy [23, 24]. The procedure can be primarily divided into the following stages: (1) Corneal Incision; (2) Capsulorhexis; (3) Phacoemulsification; and (4) Intraocular Lens (IOL) Implantation (**Figure 3**).

The management of cataracts that substantially impair vision encompasses: (1) surgical extraction of the lens material to restore an optically clear visual axis; (2) correction of the resultant aphakic refractive error using spectacles, contact lenses, or intraocular lens implantation; and (3) treatment of any concurrent sensory deprivation amblyopia.

In pediatric patients undergoing cataract removal, the use of spectacles may be impractical, rendering contact lenses a medical necessity for visual rehabilitation. Intraocular lens implantation has become a standard approach for visual rehabilitation in children aged 2 years and older [25]. Two multicenter trials [2, 26] have investigated the visual outcomes in very young children treated with either contact lenses or intraocular lens implants. One year post-treatment, children assigned to the intraocular lens implant group experienced a higher incidence of intraoperative complications, adverse events, and required additional intraocular surgeries. Although the median visual acuity was superior in the contact lens group, the difference was not statistically significant. The treatment of amblyopia remains the most challenging

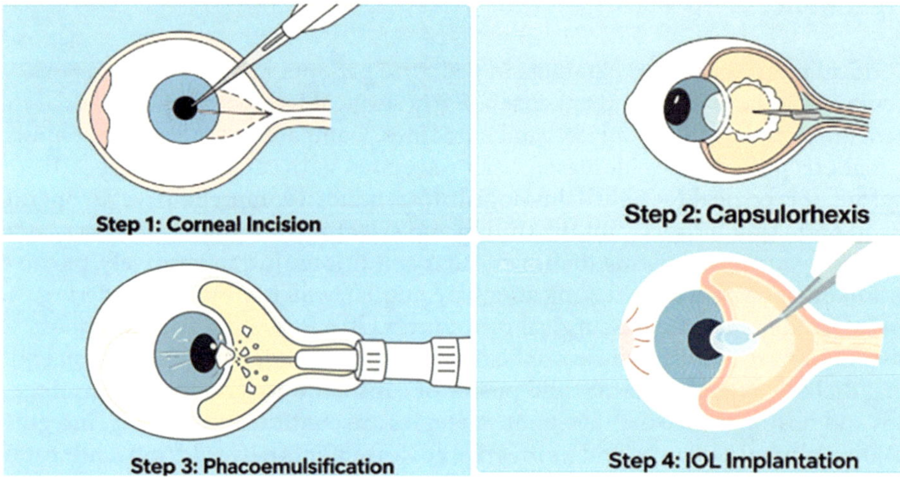

Figure 3.
Simulation diagram for pediatric cataract surgical procedure.

and demanding aspect of visual rehabilitation in infants and children with cataracts. Ophthalmic surgery remains the main treatment and is potentially beneficial for patients with diabetic cataracts, particularly after rapid and effective glycemic control (**Figure 4**) [27]. It is important to note that not all cataracts necessitate surgical intervention [28]. Cataracts that do not significantly impair vision should be regularly monitored for changes, and the child should be assessed for the development of amblyopia (**Table 1**).

5. Prognosis

The prognosis is influenced by various factors, including the characteristics of the cataract, the underlying disease, the age at onset, the age at which intervention occurs, the duration and severity of any accompanying amblyopia, and the presence of associated ocular abnormalities such as microphthalmia, retinal lesions, optic atrophy, glaucoma, nystagmus, and strabismus. Nevertheless, cataract surgery is not devoid of complications, necessitating careful consideration of the long-term risks associated with T1DM and its impact on the growth and development of the anterior eye segment [29]. The most prevalent complications following cataract surgery include posterior capsular opacification (PCO), secondary glaucoma, retinal detachment, amblyopia, and acute complications such as incision leakage, increased intraocular pressure, edema, and uveitis [30, 31]. Management of PCO differs between younger and older children, as PCO is more frequently observed in younger children. Persistent amblyopia remains the leading cause of suboptimal visual recovery post-cataract surgery in pediatric patients. In pediatric patients who have undergone cataract surgery, the development of secondary conditions and complications is possible. These may include inflammatory sequelae, secondary membrane formation, glaucoma, retinal detachment, and alterations in the axial length of the eye. It is imperative that these potential outcomes are taken into account when planning treatment strategies.

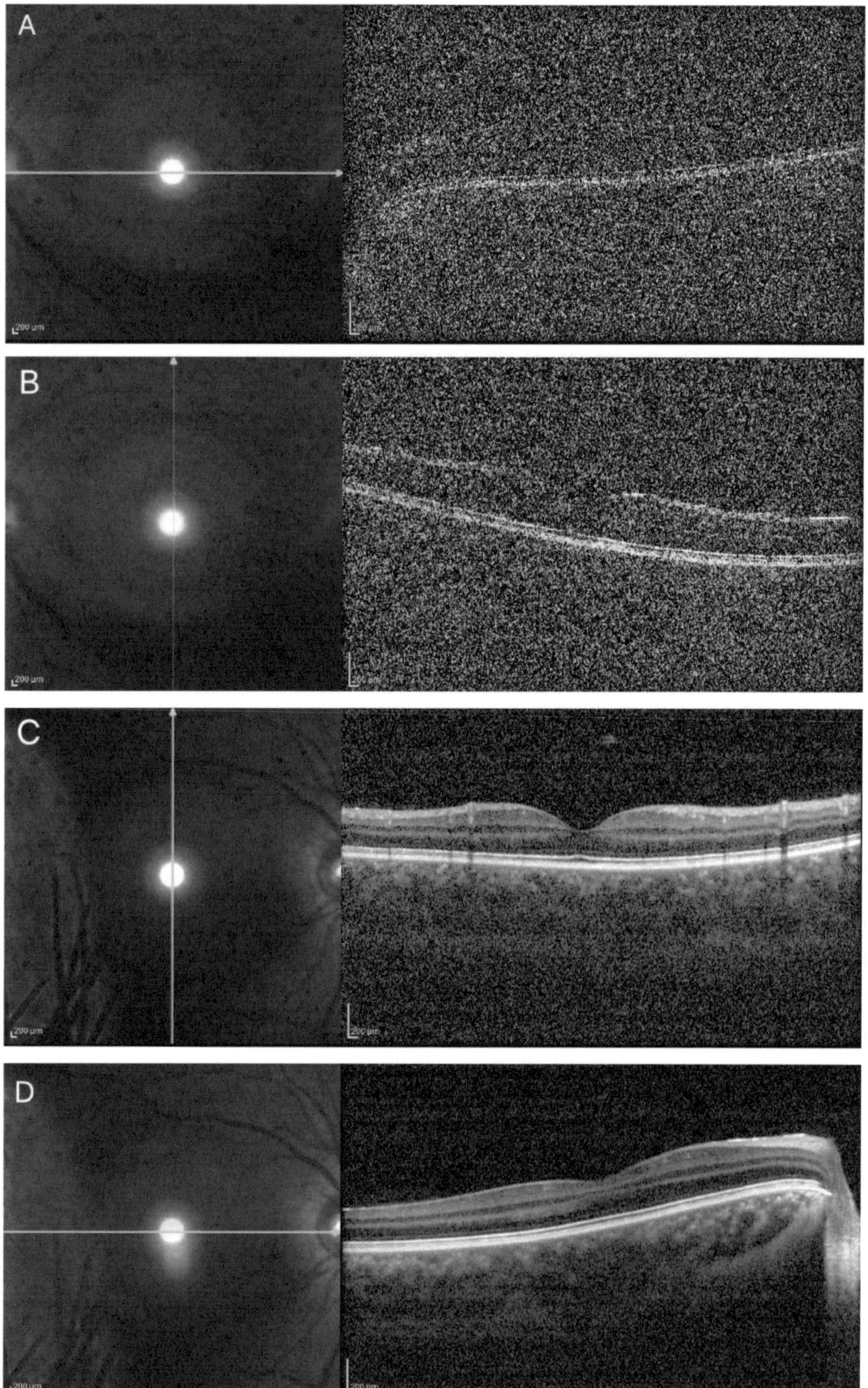

Figure 4.
Preoperative OCT of the patient with diabetic cataract.

Developmental Variants
Prematurity (Y-suture vacuoles) with or without retinopathy of prematurity
Mittendorf dot (remnant of the hyaloid artery)
Persistent pupillary membrane (remnant of embryonic lens vasculature)
Genetic Disorders
Simple Mendelian Inheritance
Autosomal dominant (most common)
Autosomal recessive
X-linked
Major Chromosomal Defects
Trisomy disorders (13, 15, 18, 21)
Turner syndrome (45X) and so on.
Endocrinopathies
Albright hereditary osteodystrophy
Hypocalcemia (hypoparathyroidism)
Hypoglycemia
Diabetes mellitus
Congenital Infections
Toxoplasmosis
Cytomegalovirus infection
Syphilis
Rubella
Perinatal herpes simplex infection
Measles (rubeola)
Poliomyelitis
Influenza
Varicella-zoster
Ocular Anomalies
Peters anomaly (corneal opacifications with iris-corneal dysgenesis)
Rieger syndrome (iris dysplasia, myotonic dystrophy)
Microphthalmia
Coloboma
Aniridia
Mesodermal dysgenesis
Norrie disease
Persistent pupillary membrane
Posterior lenticonus
Persistent fetal vasculature
Primitive hyaloid vascular system
Retinitis pigmentosa
Miscellaneous Disorders

Atopic dermatitis
Drugs (corticosteroids)
Radiation
Trauma
Juvenile idiopathic arthritis
Retinopathy of prematurity
Spherocytosis

Table 1.
Differential diagnosis of cataracts [19].

6. Future directions and emerging therapies

Emerging therapies and future research directions for pediatric cataract associated with T1DM are multifaceted, emphasizing both the enhancement of existing treatments and the development of innovative strategies. Advances in pediatric cataract surgery have integrated techniques and technologies derived from adult cataract management; however, it is recognized that pediatric cataracts necessitate distinct approaches [32]. Significant progress has been made in understanding diabetic retinopathy, a complication closely linked to cataracts. This progress includes the utilization of retinal imaging and functional analysis for the early detection of pathologies, as well as the development of therapies targeting both the neural and vascular components of the disease [33]. Future research is likely to concentrate on optimizing the timing and techniques of cataract surgery in children with type 1 diabetes and exploring the potential benefits of emerging diabetes treatments on cataract development and surgical outcomes [34]. Interdisciplinary collaboration, encompassing fields such as ophthalmology, endocrinology, and biomedical engineering, is essential for the advancement of these research domains and the translation of findings into clinical practice.

7. Conclusion

In summary, the epidemiology of pediatric cataracts in individuals with T1DM is shaped by a multitude of factors. The clinical complexities associated with managing pediatric cataracts in this patient population include the repercussions on glycemic control, the distinct characteristics inherent to pediatric cataracts, and the psychological ramifications of these conditions. These elements underscore the need for a comprehensive and individualized management strategy. The surgical treatment of cataracts in pediatric patients with T1DM demands an approach that thoroughly addresses the specific challenges faced by this demographic, with a pronounced focus on early intervention, meticulous surgical techniques, and rigorous postoperative care.

Acknowledgements

The authors are deeply grateful to these parents and their families.

Research funding

This study was supported by Hubei Province Natural Science Foundation of China (grant no. 2025AFB588).

Conflict of interest

The authors declare no conflict of interest.

Author details

Shimin Wu[1*] and Xiaoqin Yan[2]

1 Department of Pediatrics, Tongji Hospital, Tongji Medical College, Huazhong University of Science and Technology, Wuhan, China

2 Department of Ophthalmology, Tongji Hospital, Tongji Medical College, Huazhong University of Science and Technology, Wuhan, China

*Address all correspondence to: wushiminw123@sina.com

References

[1] Sayin N, Kara N, Pekel G. Ocular complications of diabetes mellitus. World Journal of Diabetes. 2015;**6**(1):92-108

[2] Šimunović M, Paradžik M, Škrabić R, Unić I, Bućan K, Škrabić V. Cataract as early ocular complication in children and adolescents with type 1 diabetes mellitus. International Journal of Endocrinology. 2018;**2018**:6763586

[3] Reiter UM, Eckert AJ, Dunstheimer D, et al. Cataract in children and adolescents with type 1 diabetes. Insights from the German/Austrian DPV registry. Pediatric Diabetes. 2022;**23**(3):362-369

[4] Geloneck MM, Forbes BJ, Shaffer J, Ying G, Binenbaum G. Ocular complications in children with diabetes mellitus. Ophthalmology. 2015;**122**(12):2457-2464

[5] Kiziltoprak H, Tekin K, Inanc M, Goker YS. Cataract in diabetes mellitus. World Journal of Diabetes. 2019;**10**(3):140-153

[6] Uspal N, Schapiro E. Cataracts as the initial manifestation of type 1 diabetes mellitus. Pediatric Emergency Care. 2011;**27**(2):132-134

[7] Libman I, Haynes A, Lyons S, et al. ISPAD clinical practice consensus guidelines 2022: Definition, epidemiology, and classification of diabetes in children and adolescents. Pediatric Diabetes. 2022;**23**(8):1160-1174

[8] Skrabic V, Ivanisevic M, Stanic R, Unic I, Bucan K, Galetovic D. Acute bilateral cataract with phacomorphic glaucoma in a girl with newly diagnosed type 1 diabetes mellitus. Journal of Pediatric Ophthalmology & Strabismus. 2010;**47**:e1-e3

[9] Goturu A, Jain N, Lewis I. Bilateral cataracts and insulin oedema in a child with type 1 diabetes mellitus. BMJ Case Reports. 2013;**2013**:bcr2012008235

[10] Snow A, Shieh B, Chang KC, et al. Aldose reductase expression as a risk factor for cataract. Chemico-Biological Interactions. 2015;**234**:247-253

[11] Guo Z, Ma X, Zhang RX, Yan H. Oxidative stress, epigenetic regulation and pathological processes of lens epithelial cells underlying diabetic cataract. Advances in Ophthalmology Practice and Research. 2023;**3**(4):180-186

[12] Thorne CA, Grey AC, Lim JC, Donaldson PJ. The synergistic effects of polyol pathway-induced oxidative and osmotic stress in the aetiology of diabetic cataracts. International Journal of Molecular Sciences. 2024;**25**(16):9042

[13] Roy B. Pathophysiological mechanisms of diabetes-induced macrovascular and microvascular complications: The role of oxidative stress. Medical Sciences (Basel). 2025;**13**(3):87

[14] Wilson ME, Levin AV, Trivedi RH, et al. Cataract associated with type-1 diabetes mellitus in the pediatric population. Journal of American Association for Pediatric Ophthalmology and Strabismus. 2007;**11**(2):162-165

[15] Costagliola C, Dell'Omo R, Prisco F, Iafusco D, Landolfo F, Parmeggiani F. Bilateral isolated acute cataracts in three newly diagnosed insulin dependent diabetes mellitus young patients. Diabetes Research and Clinical Practice. 2007;**76**(2):313-315

[16] Iafusco D, Prisco F, Romano MR, Dell'Omo R, Libondi T, Costagliola C.

Acute juvenile cataract in newly diagnosed type 1 diabetic patients: A description of six cases. Pediatric Diabetes. 2011;**12**(7):642-648

[17] Montgomery EL, Batch JA. Cataracts in insulin-dependent diabetes mellitus: Sixteen years' experience in children and adolescents. Journal of Paediatrics and Child Health. 1998;**34**(2):179-182

[18] Jin YY, Huang K, Zou CC, Liang L, Wang XM, Jin J. Reversible cataract as the presenting sign of diabetes mellitus: Report of two cases and literature review. Iranian Journal of Pediatrics. 2012;**22**(1):125-128

[19] Stanton BF, Geme III JWS, Schor NF, Behrman RE, Kliegman RM. The 21st Edition of Nelson Textbook of Pediatrics. Available from: https://www.elsevier-elibrary.com/searchresults?keyword=&option=catalog&title=&author=%20Joseph%20St.%20Geme&type=advanced

[20] Go JA, Mamalis CA, Khandelwal SS. Cataract surgery considerations for diabetic patients. Current Diabetes Reports. 2021;**21**(12):67

[21] Chinese Cataract and Refractive Surgery Society. Zhonghua Yan Ke Za Zhi. 2022;**58**(5):326-333

[22] Lenhart PD, Lambert SR. Current management of infantile cataracts. Survey of Ophthalmology. 2022;**67**(5):1476-1505

[23] Lloyd IC, Wilson ME, Trivedi RH, Biswas S, Ashworth JL, Green E, et al. Update on pediatric cataract surgery. Asia-Pacific Journal of Ophthalmology (Philadelphia). 2025;**14**(4):100229

[24] Chen SP, Woreta F, Chang DF. Cataracts: A review. Journal of the American Medical Association. 2025;**333**(23):2093-2103

[25] Al-Bakri M, Sander B, Bach-Holm D, Larsen DA, Jensen H, Kessel L. Children with congenital and childhood cataract require frequent follow-up visits and examinations in general anaesthesia: Considerations for the strain on families. Acta Ophthalmologica. 2019;**97**(8):778-783

[26] Agarkar S, Chandrasekaran A, Panicker GJ, Raman R. Cataract surgery outcomes in children and adolescents with type 1 diabetes mellitus. Journal of AAPOS. 2024;**28**(3):103926

[27] Wu S, Yan X, Wu W, Hou L, Liang Y, Luo X. Early juvenile cataract in newly diagnosed type 1 diabetic patients: A description of two cases. Journal of Pediatric Endocrinology & Metabolism. 2024;**37**(7):652-656

[28] Jin YY, Huang K, Zou CC, Liang L, Wang XM, Jin J. Reversible cataract as the presenting sign of diabetes mellitus: Report of two cases and literature review. Iranian Journal of Pediatrics (England Ed). 2012;**22**:125-128

[29] Chen D, Gong X, Xie H, Zhu XN, Li J, Zhao YE. The long-term anterior segment configuration after pediatric cataract surgery and the association with secondary glaucoma. Scientific Reports. 2017;**7**:43015

[30] Gasper C, Trivedi RH, Wilson ME. Complications of pediatric cataract surgery. Developments in Ophthalmology. 2016;**57**:69-84

[31] Ventura MC, Sampaio VV, Ventura BV, Ventura LO, Nosé W. Congenital cataract surgery with intraocular lens implantation in microphthalmic eyes: Visual outcomes and complications. Arquivos Brasileiros de Oftalmologia. 2013;**76**(4):240-243

[32] Jody N, Santana M, Rudell J. Pediatric cataract surgery: Considerations and

updates in diagnosis and management. Current Opinion in Ophthalmology. 2023;**34**(1):58-63

[33] Honasoge A, Nudleman E, Smith M, Rajagopal R. Emerging insights and interventions for diabetic retinopathy. Current Diabetes Reports. 2019;**19**(10):100

[34] Chang KC, Li L, Sanborn TM, et al. Characterization of Emodin as a therapeutic agent for diabetic cataract. Journal of Natural Products. 2016;**79**(5):1439-1444

Section 2

Refractive Cataract Surgery with Advanced Technogy

Chapter 3

Refractive Lens Exchange Indications

Araño Ferrer Jerónimo

Abstract

Refractive lens exchange (RLE) is a refractive procedure that has been used more frequently during recent years. With the improvement in technology and outcomes in cataract surgery, the possibility to offer a solution for presbyopic patients has become a great option and even patients come to clinics seeking these surgeries. In this chapter, we will review the indications of refractive lens exchange, and when is not recommended. We will review the importance of an adequate preoperative evaluation of the patient, and the studies needed to make the most accurate IOL calculation so that the patient can have the best outcome. Finally, we discuss the contraindications and when is appropriate to do surgery and when it is not.

Keywords: refractive surgery, multifocal IOL, cataract surgery, intraocular lens exchange, EDOF IOL

1. Introduction

Phacoemulsification surgery with intraocular lens (IOL) implantation is one of the most commonly performed procedure for the treatment of cataracts, aimed at improving patients' vision. Today, people seek better visual outcomes after cataract surgery, not only for distance vision but also for improved functional vision that allows them to perform daily activities more independently and without the need for spectacles. As individuals now work for more years and increasingly rely on digital devices such as computers, smartphones, and tablets, intermediate and near vision has become critically important. This shift has transformed phacoemulsification from a procedure solely for cataract treatment into a refractive surgery as well, where delivering the best possible visual outcome is essential for achieving patient satisfaction. Refractive lens exchange (RLE) has become a viable alternative for patients who are not suitable candidate for corneal refractive procedures or phakic intraocular lenses.

In 1967, Dr. Charles D. Kelman introduced phacoemulsification surgery as a less invasive, faster, and more effective method for treating cataracts [1]. Since then, the evolution of phacoemulsification has extended to new purposes.

Refractive lens exchange is defined as the removal of a clear lens for refractive purposes, with the objective to give patients more spectacle independence, either for far, near, or both visions. RLE provides a solution by replacing the clear crystalline lens with a monofocal, multifocal, or extended depth-of-focus intraocular lens to correct each refractive error. The fast diffusion of new phacoemulsification machines and better outcomes in the surgery has led to earlier RLE surgery, as many patients have higher expectations of their visual capacity [2]. The sudden increase in this procedure in recent years can raise the ethical question of its boundaries. This chapter will explore the benefits of this procedure, the adequate patient selection, and the contraindications.

2. Patient selection and evaluation

The success of RLE depends mostly on an appropriate patient selection. The main indications for a patient that wants an IOL implantation for better vision can be summarized in these main points [2, 3]:

- Moderate to high hyperopia (> + 3.00 D).
- High Myopia in patients who are not candidates for a corneal refractive procedure or Phakic IOL.
- Significant presbyopia with a desire for spectacle independence.
- Significant corneal astigmatism.

These are the first thing to consider, but most important is the patient's age. It is considered that patients should be at least 45 years of age or older to go through a RLE [2]. This will vary depending mostly in the refractive problem of each patient and the condition of the eye. It is important to consider that RLE is an elective procedure that is performed more often in younger patients that are more active and have more visual expectations after the surgery.

2.1 Preoperative evaluation

These patients need a baseline set of studies such as those patients that are having cataract surgery. It is important to know the patient's overall health to determine whether they are an optimal candidate for surgery and how existing comorbidities may affect both surgical performance and visual outcomes. Visual acuity with Snellen chart should be performed in all patients, follow by refraction of the eye [4]. The use of questionnaires is helpful to understand the patients' unconformities with its vision; there are many validated questionnaires for measuring vision-specific measures (Visual Activities Questionnaire, The Activities of Daily Vision Scale and other) [4].

Full slit lamp evaluation of the patient's eye undilated and dilated for complete examination of the retina is the next step. A complete examination of the retina and its periphery is fundamental, even more in patients with high myopia to discard any retinal lesions that can increase the risk of retinal detachment (RD). It is important to search for clinical signs of glaucoma, macular disease, pseudoexfoliation syndrome, and poorly dilating pupils that can affect the outcomes of the surgery [5].

Preoperative assessment includes biometry that can be performed using optical laser interferometry biometry, ultrasound A-scan, or optical coherence tomography [4, 5]. It is important to obtain keratometry values with either automated devices or manually [4, 5]. Corneal topography is helpful to decide if a toric IOL is indicated [5]. The use of aberrometry is essential if a multifocal or extended depth of focus IOL is being considered [5]. Retinal optical coherence tomography (OCT) should be performed in all patients to discard any macular pathologies and to understand vitreous adherence to the macula for any possible signs of traction or macular holes [5].

The decision for continuing with the RLE should be done after carefully examining all of the studies mention above and individualizing the IOL selection for each patient depending on what was found in the studies.

2.2 IOL selection and IOL calculation

The IOL selection should be individualized for each patient. In patients with high myopia the availability of minus, zero or low plus power lenses has made possible the option to always implant and IOL, which mitigates the development of posterior capsular opacification (PCO) and reduces the risk of retinal detachment [6]. Aspherical IOLs can compensate for the positive spherical aberration of the cornea to provide better outcomes; this type of IOLs is widely used because of this characteristic [7]; it is important to know the spherical aberration (SA) of the IOL for patients who have different corneal spherical aberration so that the IOL can help compensate this; it is recommended to leave a residual spherical aberration between 0.07 and 0.10 μm [7, 8].

New designs in optics in IOLs have developed rapidly in this last years; presbyopia correcting IOL designs using different refractive methods has led to have a variety of options for each individual case. Most of these IOLs use a diffractive design to achieve good near and far vision. Currently, new designs of IOLs use a refractive segmented varifocal optic; there are also trifocal diffractive IOL that have a better intermediate vision compared to those that are purely diffractive. The extended depth of focus (EDOF) IOLs achieves an elongated focus of vision by inducing negative aberration of the IOL or by the use of a pinhole principle [7].

In **Table 1** is a summary of different IOL options with its spherical aberration.

IOL calculation should be assessed for each individual case. In a systematic review by Stopyra et al. [15], Barret Universal II was the most precise vergence formula;

IOL (Model)	Type	SA Zernike (~6 mm)
Tecnis ZCB00	Monofocal Aspheric (SA -)	−0.27 um
Tecnis Symfony ZXR00	EDOF Hybrid (SA -)	~ −0.27 um
Tecnis ZMB00	Multifocal Diffractive (SA -)	~ −0.27 um
AcrySof IQ SN60WF	Monofocal Aspheric (SA -)	−0.20 um
Clareon SY60WF	Monofocal Aspheric (SA -)	−0.20 um
Akreos Adapt AO	Monofocal Neutral SA	0.00 um
EnVista MX60	Monofocal Neutral SA	0.00 um
Rayner C-flex 570C	Monofocal Spherical (SA +)	+0.10 to +0.20 um
Mini WELL Ready	EDOF Zonal SA	SA Positive/Negative Zones
LuxSmart	EDOF Zonal SA	SA Modulated

Table 1.
Different IOLs with their optical type and Spherical Aberration [9–14].

Kane and PEARL-DGS were the most accurate among the artificial intelligence-based formulas. In patients with short eyes, PEARL-DGS formula demonstrated the highest accuracy in artificial intelligence-based formulas [16]. For patients with long eyes (>26 mm), Barret Universal II showed the most accurate results [17]. In patients with previous refractive corneal surgery, Barret True-K showed the best results in patients with previous myopic and hyperopic laser refractive surgery [18, 19].

Aside of the importance of the IOL selection and IOL calculations, there are some fundamental technical principles to be conscious during RLE: during the surgery, it is important to have minimal intraoperative manipulation with microincisions, inducing the least possible surgical astigmatism; incisions should be placed over the steepest corneal meridian if possible. The surgeon should be conscious and cause minimal damage to intraocular structures and a correct IOL implantation in the capsular bag is crucial. The surgeon should have all the precautions to reduce the risk of posterior capsule opacification [6].

3. Considerations and outcomes

3.1 Myopia

Refractive lens exchange has been widely used for correcting myopia in patients who are not suitable for corneal refractive surgery [20]. This helps in having a better overview of myopic patients undergoing RLE. RLE should be considered for patients with high myopia (> – 6.00 D or axial length > 26 mm) who are not candidates for corneal refractive procedure or phakic IOLs [21]. It is important to consider the age of the patients in this group.

Studies have shown that the younger the patient is, the risk of retinal detachment increases [21]. High myopia eyes have an increased risk of RD compared to non-myopic eyes; some studies report a prevalence of RD in high myopes between 0.71% and 3.2% [21]. This prevalence increases in patients with high myopia that underwent RLE, being a total prevalence between 1.5 and 8.1% [2]. The group at higher risk is patients with an axial length more than 28 mm and below the age of 50.

The increased risk of RD in myopic patients is considered to be because of a higher incidence of predisposing retinal lesions and vitreous changes after the procedure [22]. Therefore, the importance of a thoughtful retina examination prior to the surgery.

It is important to talk about this risk with the patient before the surgery and emphasize the importance of continuous retina examinations throughout the patient's life, to be able to prevent an RD. Higher risk of choroidal neovascularization has also been described in patients with high myopia that underwent cataract surgery [23]. Even though it has been described the increased risk of RD in this group undergoing RLE, a large 2024 meta- analysis found that the incidence of RD after RLE in general was of 0.023%, compared to 0.012% in standard cataract surgery with at least a 24 month follow-up, considered to be an uncommon complication, even though it was almost twice the incidence [24]. These numbers reflect low risk, but the increase is clinically significant, especially when evaluation of surgical options for younger myopic patients. An important consideration is that postoperative YAG laser capsulotomy may further increase the risk of RD; therefore, selecting an IOL with a lower likelihood of posterior capsule opacification is crucial, like an hydrophobic sharp edge IOL [2].

RLE is an effective option to correct myopia and high myopia; with the correct evaluation of each patient, it can significantly improve quality of life and achieve optimal visual acuity outcomes [25]. RLE is indicated in patients with axial length < 26 mm who are over 50 years old, in the absence of other contraindications; patients between 45 and 50 years old can be considered for RLE if no primary refractive procedure is possible, as far as posterior vitreous detachment is demonstrated. RLE is not recommended in patients under the age of 45 and in eyes with axial length of 26 mm or more. In the presence of retinal risk factors, including extensive lattice degeneration, lacquer cracks or neovascular membrane is present in the fellow eye; surgery is contraindicated [2].

3.2 Hyperopia

Patients with hyperopia are more suitable for RLE mainly because hyperopic eyes typically have shorter axial lengths and shallower anterior chambers; this can make corneal refractive surgery or phakic IOL implantation less safe or technically unfeasible. Patients with hyperopia older than 45 years of age are good candidates for RLE; it offers a safe and effective alternative to correct both distance and near vision while preventing the onset of age-related cataracts.

With the advancement of multifocal, trifocal, and EDOF IOLs, hyperopic patients are suitable candidates for premium IOLs. These technologies offer an extended range of vision and are particularly optimal in presbyopic hyperopes who seek spectacle independence. Some recent studies have shown great patient satisfaction and quality of life following bilateral implantation of multifocal IOLs in hyperopic patients, with over 85% of patients with complete spectacle independence [26].

Another benefit is that hyperopic eyes, due to their shorter axial length and less vitreoretinal degeneration, have shown almost no incidence of RD after RLE [27]. Additionally, some hyperopic patients may have angle closure risk due to shallow anterior chamber; RLE can help deepen the anterior chamber and eliminate the potential risk of pupillary block or acute angle-closure glaucoma [28].

3.3 Astigmatism

Different approaches can be made for correcting astigmatism during RLE. Clear corneal incision in the steepest meridian is an effective way in low astigmatisms <1.00 D [29]. Another approach is to use single or paired peripheral corneal relaxing incisions that can correct astigmatisms up to 3.00 D. Nowadays, the use of toric IOLs is an effective way to correct astigmatism up to 12.00 D. Most of premium IOLs can have toricity to correct symmetric astigmatism. This helps patients to have great visual outcomes after surgery.

It is important to address astigmatism in patients with premium IOLs, because residual astigmatism can lower visual acuity and increase optical aberrations that can impact patient satisfaction and quality of vision. This reduction in quality vision is mainly due to reduced contrast sensitivity and increase in halos and glare [29, 30].

During surgery, it is critical to align the toric lens in the correct orientation for astigmatic correction, because for every 3 degrees of rotation, around 10% of the astigmatic correction is lost [7].

3.4 Presbyopia

Nowadays, presbyopia is the most common refractive error. With the increase in life expectancy, most people will live many years of their lives with presbyopia, with increasing dependence on their intermediate and near vision. Many patients that go through an RLE might be seeking more spectacle independence. RLE with premium IOLs (multifocal, trifocal, or EDOF) is one of the most common procedures for the correction of presbyopia.

When considering RLE in a patient who wants to correct presbyopia, it is important to consider their other refractive errors to address them as mention above. Patients who seek RLE for presbyopia correction and have low degrees of other refractive errors or even emmetropia with great distance vision should be address carefully about their expectations. This group of patients can have worse contrast sensitivity and more corneal aberrations after surgery that may impact their satisfaction and be very demanding on their new vision [29]. Presbyopia RLE in emmetropic patients should only be considered in the presence of advanced presbyopia [2].

4. Conclusion

Refractive lens exchange has gained more popularity among refractive procedures. It is a valid and proven method to correct refractive problems. It is important to remember that this is an elective procedure, and many of these patients can have great vision with the use of glasses or contact lenses. As physician is important to always seek for the better benefit of the patient.

In this chapter, we reviewed the importance of doing a thoughtful examination before considering an RLE. Is important to consider that all surgeries can have complications and always protecting the integrity of the person is the most ethical thing to do. RLE should be done after a good physical and ophthalmological examination, the correct analysis of the required studies performed to the patient, and, last but not the least important, after a well-informed talk with the patient.

RLE in myopic eyes is not recommended in patients under 45 years of age with axial length > 26 mm. In patients between 45 and 50 years, it should be done after ruling out any retinal comorbidities. In patients with hyperopia, it is recommended to do an RLE in those with moderate to high hyperopia, and it is not recommended in patients under 45 years of age. Finally, in patients with presbyopia and emmetropia, it should be carefully addressed and done in the presence of advanced presbyopia in an unsatisfied patient [2].

Conflict of interest

The author declares no conflict of interest.

DOI: http://dx.doi.org/10.5772/intechopen.1012886

Author details

Arañó Ferrer Jerónimo
Asociación para Evitar la Ceguera en México, Mexico City, Mexico

*Address all correspondence to: jeronimoaranof@gmail.com

References

[1] Leffler CT, Schwartz SG. How Charles Kelman invented phacoemulsification in the 1960s: A reappraisal. Heliyon. 2025;**11**(6):e42912. ISSN 2405-8440

[2] Alio JL, Pederzolli M, Grzybowski A. Refractive lens exchange: What are the red lines? European Journal of Ophthalmology. 2024;**34**:317-322. DOI: 10.1177/11206721231218909

[3] Alió JL, Grzybowski A, Romaniuk D. Refractive lens exchange in modern practice: When and when not to do it? Eye and Vision. 2014;**1**:10. DOI: 10.1186/s40662-014-0010-2

[4] American Academy of Ophthalmology Preferred Practice Pattern Cataract and Anterior Segment Panel. Cataract in the Adult Eye [Preferred Practice Pattern®]. American Academy of Ophthalmology. (USA: The Hoskins Center for Quality Eye Care). 2021. Available from: https://www.aao.org/education/preferred-practice-pattern/cataract-in-adult-eye-ppp-2021-in-press [Retrieved from: 9 July 2025]

[5] Asia Pacific Association of Cataract & Refractive Surgeons. PPP cataract surgery. Singapore, at 11 Third Hospital Avenue. 2017. Available from: https://apacrs.org/ppp_cataract_EN/files/assets/common/downloads/APACRS-PPP-Cataract%20Surgery..pdf [Retrieved: July 9, 2025]

[6] Kaweri L, Wavikar C, James E, Pandit P, Bhuta N. Review of current status of refractive lens exchange and role of dysfunctional lens index as its new indication. Indian Journal of Ophthalmology. 2020;**68**(12):2797-2803. DOI: 10.4103/ijo.IJO_2259_20

[7] Ang M, Gatinel D, Reinstein DZ, Mertens E, Alió Del Barrio JL, Alió JL. Refractive surgery beyond 2020. Eye (London, England). 2021;**35**(2):362-382. DOI: 10.1038/s41433-020-1096-5. Epub 2020 Jul 24

[8] Michael L, Kata M, Illés K, Veronika V-MP. Effect of spherical aberration on the optical quality after implantation of two different aspherical intraocular lenses. Journal of Ophthalmology. Aug; 2017:8039719, 6 pages

[9] Steinmüller LN, Greve D, Rua Amaro D, Bertelmann E, von Sonnleithner C. Analysis of higher-order aberrations in relation to the clinical outcome of an enhanced monofocal IOL. European Journal of Ophthalmology. Nov 2023;**33**(6):2096-2105. DOI: 10.1177/11206721221134171. Epub 2022 Oct 22

[10] Kim EC, Cho SY, Kang JE, Nam G, Yoon YC, Whang WJ, et al. Comparative analysis of optical quality of monofocal, enhanced monofocal, multifocal, and extended depth of focus intraocular lenses: A mobile model eye study. Translational Vision Science & Technology. 2023;**12**(7):5. DOI: 10.1167/tvst.12.7.5

[11] Karam M, Alkhowaiter N, Alkhabbaz A, Aldubaikhi A, Alsaif A, Shareef E, et al. Extended depth of focus versus trifocal for intraocular lens implantation: An updated systematic review and meta-analysis. American Journal of Ophthalmology. 2023;**251**:52-70. DOI: 10.1016/j.ajo.2023.01.024. Epub 2023 Feb 1

[12] Holladay JT. Quality of Vision: Essential Optics for the Cataract and Refractive Surgeon. Slack Incorporated; SLACK Incorporated 6900 Grove Road Thorofare, NJ 08086. USA. 2007

[13] Gharaee H, Zabihifard M, Eslampour A, Hassanzadeh S,

Shafiee M. A comparative study on visual and optical performance of Akreos AO and Kontur AB IOLs after phacoemulsification cataract surgery. Journal of Current Ophthalmology. 2016;**28**(1):12-16

[14] Charman WN. Aberrations and myopia. Ophthalmic and Physiological Optics. 2005 Jul;**25**(4):285-301. DOI: 10.1111/j.1475-1313.2005.00297.x

[15] Stopyra W, Langenbucher A, Grzybowski A. Intraocular lens power calculation formulas-a systematic review. Ophthalmology and Therapy. 2023;**12**(6):2881-2902. DOI: 10.1007/s40123-023-00799-6. Epub 2023 Sep 12

[16] Zheng X, Li M, Guo ZX, et al. Network meta-analysis of intraocular lens power calculation formulas based on artificial intelligence in short eyes. BMC Ophthalmology. 2025;**25**:225. DOI: 10.1186/s12886-025-04066-z

[17] León AA, Pierdant-Pérez M, Cámara-Miranda CB, Tirado-Aguilar RD, Esparza-Villalpando V. Fórmulas para Cálculo de lente Intraocular en Cirugía Faco Refractiva de Pacientes con Miopía alta ¿Cuál? es la más Precisa? Revisión Sistemática y Metaanálisis de la Literatura. 2023;**97**(2S):40-54

[18] Li H, Nan L, Li J, Song H. Accuracy of intraocular lens power calculation formulae after laser refractive surgery in myopic eyes: A meta-analysis. Eye and Vision (Lond). 2020;7:37. DOI: 10.1186/s40662-020-00188-1

[19] Vrijman V, Abulafia A, van der Linden JW, van der Meulen IJE, Mourits MP, Lapid-Gortzak R. ASCRS calculator formula accuracy in multifocal intraocular lens implantation in hyperopic corneal refractive laser surgery eyes. Journal of Cataract and Refractive Surgery. 2019;**45**(5):582-586. DOI: 10.1016/j.jcrs.2018.12.006. Epub 2019 Feb 28

[20] Horgan N, Condon PI, Beatty S. Refractive lens exchange in high myopia: Long term follow up. The British Journal of Ophthalmology. 2005;**89**(6):670-672. DOI: 10.1136/bjo.2004.052720

[21] Alió JL. Lens surgery (cataract and refractive lens exchange) retinal detachment risk in myopes: Still an issue? British Journal of Ophthalmology. 2011;**95**:301-303

[22] Ravalico G, Michieli C, Vattovani O, Tognetto D. Retinal detachment after cataract extraction and refractive lens exchange in highly myopic patients. Journal of Cataract and Refractive Surgery. 2003;**29**(1):39-44. DOI: 10.1016/s0886-3350(02)01508-0

[23] Hayashi K, Ohno-Matsui K, Futagami S, Ohno S, Tokoro T, Mochizuki M. Choroidal neovascularization in highly myopic eyes after cataract surgery. Japanese Journal of Ophthalmology. 2006;**50**(4):345-348. DOI: 10.1007/s10384-006-0335-z

[24] Passaro ML, Kilic D, Virgili G, Romano V, Lucenteforte E, Dick B, et al. Retinal detachment incidence in refractive lens exchange versus cataract surgery: Uncommon versus rare - systematic review and meta-analysis. The British Journal of Ophthalmology. 2025;**109**(7):756-764. DOI: 10.1136/bjo-2024-326592

[25] Srinivasan B, Leung HY, Cao H, Liu S, Chen L, Fan AH. Modern phacoemulsification and intraocular lens implantation (refractive lens exchange) is safe and effective in treating high myopia. Asia Pacific Journal of Ophthalmology (Phila). 2016;**5**(6):438-444. DOI: 10.1097/APO.0000000000000241

[26] Yim CK, Dave A, Strawn A, Chan J, Zhou I, Zhu DC. Visual outcomes and patient satisfaction after bilateral refractive lens exchange with a trifocal intraocular lens in patients with presbyopia. Ophthalmology and Therapy. 2023;**12**(3):1757-1773

[27] Clinical Gate. Refractive lens exchange. In: Clinical Ophthalmology, UK. n.d. Available from: https://clinicalgate.com/refractive-lens-exchange/ [Retrieved: July 2025]

[28] Azuara-Blanco A, Burr J, Ramsay C, Cooper D, Foster PJ, Friedman DS, et al. Effectiveness of early lens extraction for the treatment of primary angle-closure glaucoma (EAGLE): A randomised controlled trial. Lancet. 2016;**388**(10052):1389-1397. DOI: 10.1016/S0140-6736(16)30956-4

[29] Yin XL, Ji ZY, Li XX, Liang XM, Ji SX. Surgical approaches to correct corneal astigmatism at time of cataract surgery: A mini-review. International Journal of Ophthalmology. 2024;**17**(7):1370-1374. DOI: 10.18240/ijo.2024.07.23

[30] Black DA, Bala C, Alarcon A, Vilupuru S. Tolerance to refractive error with a new extended depth of focus intraocular lens. Eye (London, England). 2024;**38**(Suppl. 1):15-20. DOI: 10.1038/s41433-024-03040-1. Epub 2024 Apr 5. Erratum in: Eye (Lond). 2025;39(1):203. DOI: 10.1038/s41433-024-03422-5

Chapter 4

Advanced Techniques in Refractive Cataract Surgery (RCS): Achieving Spectacle Independence with Precision Technology

Amr Saad and Detlev R.H. Breyer

Abstract

This chapter explores the latest advancements in refractive cataract surgery (RCS), with a focus on techniques and technologies that increase spectacle independence and enhance the patient's quality of life. It provides a deep analysis of premium intraocular lenses (IOLs), including multifocal and extended depth of focus (EDOF) designs. It details their optical principles, clinical outcomes, and patient suitability. The chapter also examines the roles of corneal surgery and femtosecond laser-assisted cataract surgery (FLACS) in achieving surgical precision and optimizing refractive outcomes. These include corneal touch-up procedures such as keratorefractive lenticule extraction (KLEx, including SMILE-Pro), laser *in situ* keratomileusis (LASIK), and photorefractive keratectomy (PRK) for correcting residual refractive errors. Additionally, the chapter addresses postoperative challenges, such as dysphotopsia, reduced contrast sensitivity, light distribution, and neuroadaptation. It also highlights emerging trends, including enhanced monofocal, spiral, and pinhole IOLs. By integrating evidence-based insights with nearly two decades of practical experience in a private, premium clinical setting with scientific work and international speaking, this chapter provides ophthalmic and refractive surgeons with the knowledge necessary to optimize the patient outcomes in modern cataract surgery on an individual basis.

Keywords: refractive cataract surgery, RCS, intraocular lenses, IOL, multifocal IOL, MIOL, EDOF, extended depth of focus IOL, femtosecond laser-assisted cataract surgery, FLACS, patient selection, preoperative assessment, postoperative management, dysphotopsia, neuroadaptation

1. Introduction

Modern refractive cataract surgery has advanced significantly, expanding beyond the restoration of basic visual function to a technologically sophisticated approach that manages cloudy lens changes and addresses the entire range of refractive errors simultaneously [1]. This transformation from classic cataract surgery, which resulted in patients needing glasses after surgery, to refractive cataract surgery (RCS), which results patients being able to see without glasses, represents a fundamental reevaluation of surgical objectives. This aligns with patient lifestyle demands and is associated with the aging of the global population and the rise in patient demands [2]. In this modern era, ophthalmic surgeons must navigate a multifaceted landscape, characterized by sophisticated diagnostic modalities, diverse surgical options and devices, and complex preoperative and postoperative management strategies to achieve the optimal outcomes for each individual patient [3].

This chapter provides ophthalmologists and ophthalmic surgeons with a foundational understanding of the latest evidence-based strategies for effectively navigating this complex and rapidly evolving field. Key topics include patient selection, various intraocular lens (IOL) technologies, femtosecond laser-assisted cataract surgery (FLACS), postoperative management, and emerging trends. Supported by recent scientific literature and two decades of practical clinical experience, pioneering work, and key opinion leadership in the field of minimally invasive cataract surgery, advanced technology IOLs, and laser surgery, these topics are presented by Detlev R.H. Breyer.

1.1 Evolution of RCS

Cataract surgery has undergone a remarkable transformation, progressing from basic interventions aimed at achieving light perception to sophisticated refractive procedures designed to optimize visual performance across multiple distances. This evolution demonstrates the continuous refinement of surgical techniques and a better understanding of visual physiology, resulting in today's personalized precision-driven approach of RCS [2].

The earliest documented cases of cataract interventions date back to the fifth century BC, when couching techniques were used to displace the clouded lens into the vitreous cavity [4, 5]. These interventions were associated with severe complications, including permanent blindness. The true cataract extraction procedure was then initiated by Jacques Daviel in 1747 when he performed the first successful extracapsular cataract extraction (ECCE). This was then followed by Samuel Sharp's subsequent development of intracapsular cataract extraction (ICCE) in 1753.

The introduction of intraocular lenses (IOLs) by Sir Harold Ridley in 1949 marked the beginning of the modern era of cataract surgery and laid the foundation for refractive enhancement [6]. Ridley observed that Royal Air Force pilots could tolerate acrylic fragments in their eyes after being injured by aircraft canopies. This led him develop polymethylmethacrylate (PMMA) IOLs, which addressed the fundamental problem of aphakia and established the concept of lens replacement rather than simple removal [7]. The revolutionary implementation of ultrasonic energy-based phacoemulsification, pioneered by Charles Kelman in 1967, enabled the fragmentation of the crystalline lens through small incisions of 3 millimeters or less [8]. This approach significantly reduced surgically induced astigmatism (SIA) and accelerated visual recovery. The later development of foldable IOL materials, including silicone IOLs, was a pivotal advancement in enhancing the predictability of refractive outcomes [9].

The twenty-first century brought further advancements in surgical precision and IOL technology, transforming cataract surgery into a refractive procedure capable of addressing the entire spectrum of ametropia. The introduction of FLACS in 2008 represented a paradigm shift toward more automated and predictable surgical precision. FLACS enables reproducible capsulotomies, precise lens fragmentation, and accurate corneal incisions [10]. Trifocal or multifocal IOLs (MIOLs) can provide functional vision at near, intermediate, and distance ranges, whereas extended depth of focus (EDOF) lenses use novel optical designs to extend the range of clear vision while minimizing the optical phenomena associated with traditional MIOL designs [11, 12]. Recent advancements include light-adjustable, spiral, and accommodative IOLs [13].

1.2 Today's paradigm shift

The modern transformation of RCS encompasses technological advancements and patient-centered approaches. Historically, the rationale for cataract surgery has been limited to cases of visually significant cataracts. The efficacy of this surgical intervention has predominantly been assessed based on enhancing distance visual acuity (VA) and reducing glare. The timing of surgery was typically based on cataract density and its impact on daily activities.

Modern RCS takes a proactive and comprehensive approach to intervention, considering lens replacement as an opportunity for visual enhancement rather than simply cataract treatment. This requires modified, comprehensive patient selection criteria that include multifactorial assessment protocols extending beyond traditional clinical parameters to encompass lifestyle demands, visual requirements, and psychosocial factors (see Chapter 2.2).

The integration of advanced diagnostic and surgical technologies has enabled unprecedented precision in surgical interventions and customized treatment protocols. Artificial intelligence (AI) algorithms that enhance the accuracy of intraocular lens (IOL) power calculations, such as the Hill-RBF and Pearl-DGS methods, are continuously refined based on real-world outcome data [14, 15]. These algorithms are particularly beneficial for eyes with atypical dimensions or a history of refractive surgery, where accurately calculating the IOL power is challenging.

1.3 Core principles of RCS

Successful RCS is founded on three interconnected pillars that collectively determine surgical outcomes: precise preoperative assessment and planning with the most up-to-date diagnostics and an experienced team, careful intraoperative execution by an experienced, high-volume surgeon, and comprehensive postoperative management including touch-up surgery in 5–10% of cases. It is important to understand that RCS operates within significantly narrower tolerance margins compared to conventional cataract surgery. Even minor deviations in planning or execution can substantially impact final refractive outcomes and patient satisfaction, so it should only be performed by experienced, high-volume surgeons in a premium setting.

2. Patient selection and preoperative assessment

2.1 Preoperative evaluation of potential RCS candidates

A comprehensive preoperative evaluation is essential for achieving successful outcomes in RCS. This process integrates multimodal diagnostics to evaluate the ocular surface, corneal structure, biometric parameters, posterior segment health, and systemic factors to minimize refractive surprises and optimize patient satisfaction [3].

A thorough medical history is the cornerstone of the preoperative assessment in RCS. It helps identify potential risk factors and contraindications, thereby decreasing the likelihood of complications [3]. Key elements include a review of current medications. For example, alpha-1 adrenergic blockers (e.g., tamsulosin) increase the risk of intraoperative floppy iris syndrome (IFIS) [16]. Hereditary eye conditions, such as keratoconus (KC) or glaucoma, could also lead to poor RCS outcomes [17, 18]. The ocular history should include any prior surgeries, such as photorefractive keratectomy, as well as any history of trauma or maculopathies. These factors can increase higher-order aberrations (HOAs) and limit visual outcomes with MIOLs [19]. A thorough systemic history is essential to identifying comorbidities that could impair healing or outcomes. For example, diabetes mellitus increases the risk of postoperative cystoid macular edema (CME) [20]. Lifestyle and daily activities (e.g., hobbies, night driving, screen-based work) should be explored in depth to tailor IOL selection to the patient's functional demands [21]. Patients who frequently drive at night are better candidates for EDOF IOLs rather than diffractive MIOLs because the latter can worsen photopsias like halos and glare in low-light (mesopic) conditions, which can lead to reduced vision [22].

The clinical examination is a multifaceted process that aims to comprehensively evaluate ocular health and identify pathologies that could compromise surgical success [3]. Beginning with the anterior segment, slit-lamp biomicroscopy is essential for evaluating corneal clarity and excluding corneal degenerations and dystrophies, including epithelial or stromal opacities, and endothelial guttata, which may indicate Fuchs' endothelial corneal dystrophy, which holds the risk of postoperative corneal decompensation. Assessing pupil size under mesopic (dim light) and photopic (bright light) conditions is crucial especially for MIOL candidates. Small pupils in mesopic settings can impair near vision in pupil-dependent MIOL designs, while large pupils in photopic settings can exacerbate halos and glare [23]. Angle kappa (κ) measurements are critical because values exceeding 0.5 mm have been associated with an increased risk of dysphotopsia and reduced VA in MIOL patients, although the evidence is mixed [24, 25]. Determining ocular dominance, typically done *via* the hole-in-card test, is vital for allocating the motoric dominant eye to distance correction in blended vision approaches and accelerating postoperative neuroadaptation [26]. Another valuable test for determining the dominant eye is to blur the vision with a + 1.0 diopter (D) lens and ask the patient which eye is more distracting. Never forget to ask the patient which eye he uses to shoot a rifle. Due to its high prevalence, which is often exacerbated by age-related meibomian gland dysfunction (MGD), assessing dry eye disease (DED) assessment is essential [27]. Using the Ocular Surface Disease Index (OSDI) questionnaire to quantify symptoms can inform preoperative management decisions, including intense pulsed light therapy with meibomian gland expression (IPL-MGX) or thermal pulsation systems (e.g., LipiFlow) [28]. A dilated fundus examination is essential for identifying retinal pathologies, such as age-related macular degeneration (AMD), epiretinal membranes (ERM), and peripheral degenerations predisposing to retinal detachment (RD), particularly in myopic eyes. A detached vitreous should be documented. Although retinal diseases are often considered relative contraindications for Advanced Technology (AT) IOLs, recent evolving analyses suggest that mild, stable conditions may not preclude AT-IOL use. Objective (autorefractor) and subjective (phoropter) refractions, along with distance and near VA and contrast sensitivity testing, establish fundamental baseline RCS metrics.

Finally, biometry and high-resolution imaging form the technical foundation of the preoperative evaluation in RCS [3]. These technologies are used to precisely calculate and select the IOL power and to identify subtle anatomical variations that could significantly influence outcomes. Prior to these assessments, patients must stop wearing contact lenses (CL) for at least 14 days to avoid lens-induced corneal distortion and inaccurate IOL calculations [29]. Aberrometry is essential for measuring HOAs, such as spherical aberration (SA). High corneal HOA values often contraindicate MIOL implantation and guide surgeons toward monofocal or EDOF alternatives. Precise axial length (AL) measurement *via* optical biometry (e.g., IOLMaster or Lenstar) is critical for IOL power calculations. Eyes with high myopia (AL >26 mm) require caution due to an increased risk of RD postoperatively, so patients need thorough education. Scheimpflug tomography (e.g., Pentacam), combined with biomechanical analysis *via* Corvis ST, assesses corneal hysteresis and resistance. This helps to exclude subclinical KC through parameters such as the tomographic-biomechanical index (TBI). Corneal pachymetry can map central and peripheral thickness. Thin corneas pose a heightened risk of ectasia in potential touch-up procedures like LASIK and should be excluded [30]. Additionally, endothelial cell density measured by specular microscopy is essential for evaluating decompensation risk [31]. Irregular astigmatism patterns, such as skewed axes or asymmetry, as measured by keratometry and topography, contraindicate MIOL implantation due to the reduced predictability. In general, targeting postoperative astigmatism of less than 0.75 D is key for AT-IOL efficacy. Lastly, retinal OCT imaging can rule out pathologies such as epiretinal membranes or early CME precursors and optic nerve damage.

2.2 Patient selection and preoperative counseling in RCS

Ideal candidates for RCS are generally healthy individuals with active lifestyles who are motivated to achieve independence from glasses and have realistic expectations about surgical outcomes. Accurate IOL power calculations and predictable outcomes depend on refractive stability. Ideal candidates should demonstrate this stability over at least 2 years. Age is also a key factor, as optimal candidates are typically 40 years or older to balance the need for presbyopia correction with the elevated risk of retinal detachment in younger patients [32]. We do not recommend clear lens exchange solely for optical reasons and only perform lens surgery on cloudy crystalline lenses. Otherwise, we prefer corneal or ICL surgery to avoid the higher complication rate inherent to IOL surgery.

Success in RCS depends on aligning patient expectations with the achievable outcomes. Candidates must understand potential trade-offs, such as glare or halos with MIOLs, and accept that they may need glasses for certain activities. Completely eliminating the need for glasses is (currently) unrealistic and technically impossible. It is crucial to explicitly address visual expectations, including the desire for spectacle independence, as unrealistic expectations significantly contribute to IOL explanations. The difference should be explained to the patient as achievable spectacle independence versus unrealistic freedom from spectacles. In this context, screening for personality traits such as perfectionism, anxiety, and depression is essential. Tools like the Five Factor Inventory (FFI) scale can assess these traits, which are linked to an increased risk of dissatisfaction, even following technically successful surgery [33]. A history of nonadherence to postoperative care regimens signals unsuitability because diligence in follow-up care is nonnegotiable.

The efficacy of RCS procedures depends heavily on comprehensive patient education and counseling. This counseling should include translating complex optical principles into the understandable concepts [34, 35]. Nowadays, patients have a growing number of options for independent education before to undergoing refractive surgery, which makes overcoming prejudiced opinions more challenging. RCS is based on shared decision-making, a collaborative approach that enables patients to actively participate in selecting an IOL and surgical plan that align to their unique visual needs and lifestyle preferences [36]. The informed consent process must explicitly outline these factors to ensure that patients understand the full scope of the procedure, including the potential need for additional interventions to refine their vision. To enhance comprehension, clinicians may use visual aids or IOL simulators to illustrate how different IOLs might affect postoperative vision and to preview potential visual outcomes with multifocal or EDOF IOLs and anticipate phenomena like glare or halos [37]. Transparency regarding the financial and legal aspects of RCS is critical for making an informed decision. Patients should receive a clear explanation of the differences between standard cataract surgery, which is usually covered by insurance, and RCS options, which often require additional out-of-pocket payments.

Regardless of patient suitability, it is important to note that integrating RCS into conventional ophthalmological practice requires considering surgical training requirements, capital expenditures on specialized equipment, and workflow modifications (e.g., increased counseling time). Therefore, it may not be applicable to all practices or clinics.

3. Multifocal intraocular lenses (MIOLs)

3.1 Optical principles and design

Multifocal intraocular lenses (MIOLs) represent a significant advancement in presbyopia-correcting IOL technology. Diffractive MIOLs enable functional vision across far, intermediate, and near distances by simultaneously projecting multiple focal points onto the retina [38]. Unlike monofocal IOLs, which provide a single focal point and typically require additional correction for near or intermediate vision, diffractive MIOLs distribute incoming light to generate overlapping depth-of-focus (DOF) zones. However, this optical strategy introduces inherent trade-offs, including reduced contrast sensitivity and photopic phenomena such as halos and glare. These phenomena arise from unfocused light rays and neural processing challenges [39].

The foundational principle of MIOLs is the manipulation of light through refraction, diffraction, or hybrid mechanisms [40]. First refractive MIOLs use variations in lens curvature or zonal power to bend light rays differently across the optic surface. Early designs, introduced in the 1990s, featured concentric or annular zones with distinct refractive powers and often incorporated a near addition of +3.0 to +4.0 diopters (D) [41]. For example, the central zones were optimized for distance vision, and the peripheral zones focused light for near tasks. This zonal refraction created discrete foci but was highly dependent on the pupil size. Optimal visual performance required a mesopic pupil diameter of approximately 3–4 mm to evenly distribute light distribution evenly between zones. However, the abrupt transitions between zones led to light scattering and edge effects, resulting in halos and glare. This limited their widespread adoption despite their ability to provide good near and far vision [42].

To address these limitations, diffractive optics emerged. First introduced in 1987 with models like the 815E/815X (3 M, now discontinued), these lenses use microscopic echelettes, or step-like gratings etched onto the lens surface, to split incoming light into multiple diffraction orders [43]. The zeroth order typically directs light to the distance focus, while the first order creates the near focus [44]. Trifocal diffractive designs, such as the AcrySof IQ PanOptix (Alcon) and the AT LISA tri (Carl Zeiss Meditec), introduce an intermediate focus, with an effective add power ranging from +1.66 to +2.17 D [45]. This elongates the DOF for seamless vision from approximately 40 cm to infinity. Apodization further improves this performance by gradually reducing the height of the echelettes from the center to the periphery. This directs more light to the distance focus under photopic conditions and mitigates photopic phenomena [46].

Segmental refractive designs are an alternative to concentric zoning, reducing pupil dependency and photic effects. The Lentis Mplus series (Teleon), for example, incorporates an asymmetrical inferior sector with a near addition ranging from +1.5 to +3.0 D. This design distributes light unevenly between near and distance vision [47]. While this minimizes edge-induced scatter and enhances contrast sensitivity, slight anisometropia can be induced in bilateral implantation.

Hybrid MIOLs combine the refractive and diffractive elements to leverage the strengths of both. For example the TECNIS Synergy (Johnson & Johnson Vision) that uses diffractive echelettes for multifocality and refractive asphericity to increase the DOF, resulting in high light efficiency and reduced halos [48]. Similarly, the FineVision Triumf (PhysIOL) uses a trifocal diffractive pattern with variable step heights to optimize intermediate vision and counteract corneal SA [49]. Aspheric surfaces often correct −0.20 μm of SA, which neutralizes the cornea's inherent positive SA (+0.27 μm on average). This improves contrast sensitivity and reduces coma-like aberrations.

3.2 Clinical outcomes

Recent meta-analyses consistently show that diffractive MIOLs outperform monofocal lenses in achieving uncorrected near and intermediate visual acuity. Diffractive trifocal designs have high spectacle independence rates, though they slightly reduce contrast sensitivity and increase dysphotopsia in some patients [50, 51]. These outcomes vary by optical design. Refractive MIOLs often prioritize distance and intermediate vision, while diffractive models excel in near VA [52]. Neuroadaptation, which typically resolves within 3 to 6 months, plays a critical role in subjective satisfaction [53].

Bifocal refractive MIOLs have demonstrated reliable distance VA (typically 20/20 or better uncorrected) and functional near vision in clinical trials. However, intermediate performance remains a limitation [54]. Segmental variants, such as the Lentis Mplus (Teleon), deliver better results, providing high VA at all working distances and offering spectacle independence for daily activities in up to 100% of patients [55, 56]. Patient satisfaction scores average 9/10 and are attributed to lower photic phenomena and preserved contrast sensitivity. However, slight anisometropia in bilateral implantation can necessitate a longer period of adaptation [55].

Diffractive bifocal MIOLs provide superior near VA, but at the expense of intermediate vision and visual quality. For example, the TECNIS ZMB00 (Johnson & Johnson Vision) yields an uncorrected near visual acuity of 0.10 logMAR in clinical trials. Defocus curves show a bimodal peak, and the lens provides complete spectacle independence in approximately 80% of patients [57, 58]. However, studies have highlighted a reduction in contrast sensitivity loss and the incidence of photic disturbances, which often partially resolve through neuroadaptation [59, 60]. Comparative studies against refractive bifocals indicate that diffractive models offer similar near and distance performance with high overall satisfaction rates of 9/10 [61, 62].

Trifocal diffractive MIOLs address the intermediate vision limitations of bifocals by providing smoother defocus curves from 40 cm to infinity and comparable or higher levels of spectacle independence [63]. For instance, clinical data indicate that the AcrySof IQ PanOptix (Alcon) provides UDVA of 0.01 logMAR, intermediate VA at 60 cm of 0.06 logMAR, and near VA at 40 cm of 0.04 logMAR. Over 90% of patients achieve spectacle independence, and satisfaction scores exceed 90% [64, 65]. Photopic phenomena occur more often with trifocals than with EDOF IOLs but are potentially milder than in bifocals due to optimized light distribution. Contrast sensitivity usually also dips slightly in mesopic conditions. Similarly, the AT LISA tri 839MP (Carl Zeiss Meditec) shows comparable results with an UNVA of approximately 0.16 logRAD, around 88% spectacle-free rates, and high satisfaction (over 90%). Defocus curves reveal minimal intermediate dips [66, 67]. Head-to-head comparisons with bifocal diffractive lenses confirm trifocals' superiority in intermediate VA and overall visual range, though photopsia rates are similar [57, 63].

Hybrid MIOLs, which integrate refractive and diffractive elements, often yield the highest patient-reported metrics [68, 69]. The TECNIS Synergy (Johnson & Johnson Vision) stands out in this regard, with clinical evaluations demonstrating UDVA, UIVA, and UNVA ranging from 0.00 to 0.03 logMAR. Ninety percent of patients are spectacle-independent, and satisfaction rates exceed 90% [68–70]. Photic phenomena affect less than 5% of patients, which is lower than with pure diffractive designs due to refractive smoothing. The spiral MIOL mentioned in Chapter 5.3 seems to reduce the induction of photopic phenomena even further and does not cause light loss.

4. Extended Depth of Focus (EDOF) IOLs

4.1 Optical principles and design

Extended Depth of Focus (EDOF) IOLs offer a balanced solution that addresses the limitations of both monofocal and multifocal IOL designs [71, 72]. While diffractive MIOLs achieve spectacle independence at multiple distances through discrete focal points, this is often at the expense of reduced contrast sensitivity and increased photic phenomena, such as halos and glare. Clinically, patients realize the light distribution of diffractive MIOLs in different foci, like far (60%), intermediate (30%), and near (10%) and may experience difficulty reading in mesopic conditions. In contrast, EDOF IOLs extend the focal range, enhancing intermediate and sometimes functional near vision without the significant optical compromises of traditional diffractive multifocality.

The basic optical concept behind EDOF IOLs is to adjust the incoming light to create a wider DOF than the single focal plane typical of monofocal IOLs [71]. DOF refers to the range of distances at which an image remains acceptably sharp without accommodation. These IOLs typically extend DOF by 1.5 to 2.5 D without splitting light into multiple discrete foci. This elongation reduces defocus blur and dysphotopsia, which are key challenges in presbyopia correction. EDOF IOLs provide functional vision from distance to intermediate ranges (typically 60–80 cm) and sometimes extend to near tasks (around 40–50 cm), depending on the specific IOL design [73]. EDOF IOLs use various optical strategies to achieve this DOF. They often incorporate negative aspheric surfaces to neutralize corneal SA, which typically ranges from −0.1 to −0.27 μm [74]. These strategies fall under three categories: refractive, diffractive, and minimally diffractive.

Refractive EDOF IOLs create zonal variations in power and distribute light asymmetrically and progressively across the lens optic [71, 75]. Segmental or progressive zonal optics incorporate low-add segments, typically +1.5 D, which provide intermediate vision while blending seamlessly with the distance zone. This asymmetry extends the focal range by inducing controlled defocus gradients, thereby achieving high light efficiency and reducing pupil dependency [75]. The result is an elongated focus that supports activities such as computer work or driving with minimal energy loss to HOAs.

In contrast, diffractive EDOF designs use subtle microstructural patterns, such as echelettes (low-profile diffractive gratings), to extend focus through controlled light interference [71, 76]. Unlike traditional diffractive MIOLs, which have pronounced rings that split light and lead to significant energy loss, EDOF designs aim to cause minimal diffraction. This limits light scattering and directs most energy into an elongated primary focus. This "stretched" focal zone, rather than discrete points, improves intermediate vision while reducing unwanted diffraction orders that may cause photopic phenomena. Further improvement can be achieved through aspheric integration, which modulates wavefront curvature.

Damien Gatinel coined the term minimal diffractive IOL designs, which eliminate the need for severe gratings. Instead, they use wavefront shaping or small-aperture optics to extend DOF [77–79]. Wavefront extension uses surface modifications to elongate the focal point with few diffractive elements. This further minimizes dysphotopsia while preserving contrast sensitivity. Small-aperture designs, such as the pinhole principle, use an embedded mask with a small aperture (e.g., 1.36 mm) to block peripheral rays [80]. This enhances the DOF by increasing the f-stop equivalent, similar to camera optics. However, this approach may slightly reduce light transmission and requires careful patient selection to prevent unwanted dimming in low-light conditions. Therefore, minimal diffractive EDOF IOLs are an interesting compromise between refractive and diffractive EDOF IOLs. For this reason, Detlev Breyer no longer uses diffractive EDOF IOLs but prefers refractive, segmental, and minimally diffractive EDOF IOLs.

4.2 Clinical outcomes

EDOF IOLs generally demonstrate superior intermediate VA compared to monofocal designs. Their functional near vision surpasses monofocals, though it falls short to trifocal MIOLs. EDOF IOLs present a reasonable dysphotopsia profile, comparable to monofocals [72, 81, 82]. Overall, EDOF IOLs achieve high patient satisfaction rates and high spectacle independence for intermediate tasks. However, reading glasses are commonly needed for fine near work in these patient populations [83].

On the one hand, refractive EDOF IOLs, such as the Lentis Comfort (Teleon Surgical), which integrates a + 1.5D low-add sector, have shown robust clinical results in multiple studies [84–86]. A prospective multicenter trial involving 120 eyes reported a mean binocular uncorrected intermediate VA (UIVA) of 0.1 logMAR at 70 cm. Distance VA (UDVA) was 0.00 logMAR, and near VA (UNVA) was 0.48 logMAR at 30 cm. These results indicate functional, but not full, spectacle independence for close tasks [84]. Defocus curves revealed a broad plateau from 0.00 to −1.50 D, with a VA of 20/25 or better across this range. Contrast sensitivity remained comparable to that of monofocal IOLs under the photopic conditions [85]. Dysphotopsia rates were low, with only a small percentage of patients experiencing halos and glare as also experienced with monofocal IOL, and no severe symptoms. This contributed to the satisfaction scores above 90%. The LuxSmart IOL (Bausch and Lomb) is a non-diffractive, hydrophobic acrylic EDOF lens that uses Pure Refractive Optics (PRO) technology to provide a continuous range of vision. It emphasizes intermediate distances while maintaining high contrast sensitivity and low dysphotopsia rates. Its aberration-neutral design balances the distance and intermediate VA, and clinical studies have demonstrated its superior uncorrected intermediate VA compared to monofocal lenses and its reduced halos compared to the diffractive MIOLs [87]. When used in mini-monovision (with a target of −0.50 D in the non-dominant eye), near visual acuity extends to 0.12 logMAR at 40 cm [88].

On the other hand, large-scale trials have evaluated diffractive EDOF IOLs, such as the TECNIS Symfony (Johnson & Johnson Vision), a diffractive IOL model. These trials include the Concerto study, which examined 411 eyes. The mean UDVA was −0.02

logMAR, the UIVA was 0.1 logMAR at 70 cm, and the UNVA was 0.16 logMAR at 40 cm [89]. Binocular defocus curves showed a continuous range from 0.00 to −1.50 D with VA of 0.02 logMAR or better. This performance surpassed that of monofocal IOLs in the intermediate vision range [73]. Contrast sensitivity was slightly reduced compared to aspheric monofocal IOLs, and photic phenomena were moderate [90]. A meta-analysis of five studies (466 eyes) confirmed 90% spectacle independence for daily activities and improvements in quality of life (QoL) *via* validated questionnaires like the VF-14 [91]. Another diffractive EDOF with chromatic aberration correction, the AT LARA 829MP (Carl Zeiss Meditec), mirrored these results in a comparative trial of 211 patients, achieving UIVA of 0.07 logMAR and a defocus range of to −1.5 D [92]. However, near VA lagged, necessitating glasses for reading in some patients, though dysphotopsia was low due to smoother echelette transitions.

There is strong evidence from clinical studies supporting minimally diffractive EDOF IOLs, such as the AcrySof IQ Vivity (Alcon), which employs wavefront-shaping technology for wavefront extension. These studies report UDVA of approximately 0.04 logMAR, UIVA of 0.06 logMAR at 66 cm, and UNVA of 0.21 logMAR at 40 cm [93, 94]. Defocus curves exhibited a plateau from 0.00 to −1.5 D, with binocular summation enhancing intermediate performance. Contrast sensitivity levels matched those of monofocal lenses (1.6–1.9 logCS photopically), and dysphotopsia was minimal. These results led to high patient satisfaction and 94% spectacle independence for daily activities. One study compared the Vivity IOL to trifocal MIOLs and found equivalent intermediate VA but superior contrast sensitivity and fewer visual disturbances [95]. The IC-8 Apthera (Bausch + Lomb) is a small-aperture, non-diffractive design with a 3.23 mm optic and a 1.36 mm mask. It extends the DOF *via* the pinhole effect and yields UDVA of −0.01 logMAR, UIVA of 0.05 logMAR, and functional near VA of 0.19 logMAR with the bilateral implantation [96].

4.3 EDOF blended vision: The Duesseldorf formula

In 2010, Detlev Breyer published his initial findings on the implantation of this IOL in a blended vision mode, targeting the far dominant eye for distance (emmetropia) and the non-dominant eye for −1.5 D [97]. This approach yielded excellent distance vision, very good intermediate vision, and sufficient near vision for reading print in book and newspapers [83, 98]. He also demonstrated that, after a neuroadaptation period of 1 to 3 months, 3D stereopsis returned. In the following years, he demonstrated that blended vision is an interesting option for patients seeking independence from glasses and wanting to avoid the disadvantages of diffractive MIOLs, such as photopic phenomena and reduced contrast sensitivity. Note that the Duesseldorf Formula only works with refractive and minimal diffractive EDOF IOLs, as diffractive EDOF IOLs cause too much photopic phenomena and blurry vision when defocused to −1.5D [39].

5. Emerging trends and innovations

5.1 Enhanced monofocal IOLs

Enhanced monofocal IOLs represent a hybrid approach that extends the DOF beyond that of traditional monofocal designs while preserving high contrast sensitivity and minimizing dysphotopsia [99, 100]. These lenses provide the modest extension of focus, typically improving intermediate vision at distances of around 66 cm. The

Tecnis Eyhance (Johnson & Johnson Vision), for example, has a higher-order aspheric surface that creates a continuous power progression from the center to the periphery of the optic, shifting the focal point slightly anteriorly and extending the DOF by 0.5–1.0 D compared to standard monofocal IOLs [101, 102]. This enables better uncorrected intermediate VA while maintaining distance VA [103]. The RayOne EMV (Rayner) uses a patented non-diffractive optic with positive SA to extend the DOF by up to 1.5D [104–107]. These IOLs are ideal for individuals who rely on good intermediate vision for activities such as computer work and who are wary of MIOL-related optical side effects [106]. However, the challenges of such optics include limited near distance VA, which often necessitates reading glasses for fine print, as well as variability in outcomes based on individual corneal aberrations. Detlev Breyer uses the Rayner One EMV IOL as an EDOF IOL with the Duesseldorf Formula in a blended vision mode, as the monocular and binocular defocus curves reflect typical EDOF defocus curves.

5.2 Accommodative IOLs

Accommodative IOLs aim to replicate the natural lens' ability to change focus through ciliary muscle contraction to overcome the fixed focal point principle of MIOLs or EDOF IOLs [108, 109]. These designs are usually based on shape-changing optics or anterior-posterior optic shifts. For instance, the FluidVision (Alcon, in development) uses fluid redistribution within the IOL haptics to alter the optic curvature. The Juvene (LensGen) uses a modular, fluid-filled system that can theoretically provide functional accommodation [110, 111]. However, the long-term efficacy of these IOL designs is limited and many may only provide pseudoaccommodation (e.g., *via* miosis or residual astigmatism), rather than true dynamic focus [108]. Additionally, accommodation amplitudes typically decrease over time due to capsular fibrosis or haptic fatigue.

The AkkoLens Lumina is one of the most promising accommodating IOLs, which is a sulcus-based accommodative IOL and uses the Alvarez principle and two optical elements that shift laterally during ciliary muscle contraction [112–114]. This shift alters the IOL's refractive power dynamically, providing true accommodation. Unlike capsular bag-dependent IOLs, its sulcus placement minimizes fibrosis-related complications and enhances long-term stability. A one-year, multicenter, phase III clinical trial demonstrated stable visual outcomes, including a mean uncorrected distance visual acuity (VA) of −0.01 logMAR, preserved contrast sensitivity, and an accommodative performance of −0.65 D.

5.3 Spiral IOLs

The spiral Galaxy MIOL by Rayner is an innovative presbyopia-correcting IOL that uses unconventional optic geometries to achieve DOF while minimizing common drawbacks like dysphotopsia [115]. These IOLs create progressive focus elongation through a helical refractive profile, providing smoother visual transitions across distances [116]. The RayOne Galaxy IOL (Rayner), which uses proprietary AI algorithms trained on extensive patient outcome data, was launched in Europe in 2024. It is a non-diffractive IOL with a patented spiral optic that provides a full, continuous range of vision, without the light energy loss typical of diffractive trifocal IOLs. Initial patient satisfaction metrics suggest the high levels of spectacle independence for daily activities [117].

From October 2024 to August 2025, Detlev Breyer implanted over 200 IOLs of this type. His first clinical results showed binocular defocus curves that closely resembled the Duesseldorf Formula blended vision EDOF IOL concept, offering excellent far and intermediate vision, as well as the ability to easily read book and newspaper print. Both approaches demonstrate significantly reduced photopic phenomena compared to diffractive MIOLs, with less light loss and better contrast sensitivity. The Duesseldorf Formula concept seems to be slightly more advantageous for patients who rely on excellent distance vision, such as hunters and snipers.

5.4 Further IOL innovations

Light-adjustable IOLs, such as the RxSight LAL, allow for postoperative UV light adjustments of up to ±2.0D of sphere and up to −2.0D of cylinder in multiple sessions [118]. These adjustments achieve a residual refractive error ± 1.00 D in 100% of eyes in a retrospective case series. However, they require patient compliance with light exposure restrictions [119, 120]. Modular IOL systems, like the Harmoni (ClarVista), enable optic exchange without the need for full IOL removal [121]. This could be promising for younger patients or those at risk of future retinal issues. New hydrogel materials and drug-eluting coatings could reduce posterior capsule opacification (PCO) rates and aim to extend IOL longevity [122, 123].

6. Laser surgery, refractive enhancements, and neuroadaptation

6.1 Femtosecond laser-assisted cataract surgery (FLACS)

In modern cataract extraction, femtosecond laser-assisted cataract surgery (FLACS) has emerged as a transformative advancement [10]. First introduced clinically in 2009 with the LenSx platform (Alcon Laboratories), FLACS uses femtosecond lasers that deliver pulses in the range of 10^{-15} sec, to create tissue photodisruption with minimal collateral thermal damage, achieving submicron accuracy [124]. In 2009, Detlev Breyer began using the same system but switched to the LENSAR FLACS system 1 year later because the Scheimpflug technology in the LENSAR system created free-floating buttons in a more reliable manner.

This technology is nowadays available on platforms such as the Catalys (Johnson & Johnson Vision), the Victus (Bausch + Lomb), and the Femto LDV Z8 (Ziemer Ophthalmic Systems), and it allows for optimal IOL positioning and astigmatic control [125]. The automated steps include corneal incisions, capsulotomy, and lens fragmentation. These systems improve reproducibility by reducing surgeon variability. However, its adoption remains selective due to cost issues.

In 2024, Detlev Breyer began using the newest LENSAR ALLY FLACS system, which uses innovative computer systems and multiple Scheimpflug cameras to significantly improve precision, individual settings, and speed. With this laser system, creation of the clear corneal incision (CCI) takes only 1 second, and the overall laser time can be reduced to less than 1 minute, further improving the safety and patient comfort of FLACS.

FLACS uses real-time imaging *via* integrated OCT or Scheimpflug systems to customize procedure planning based on lens density and corneal thickness [126, 127]. The primary steps include creating CCIs, performing an anterior capsulotomy, and fragmenting the lens. CCIs can be tailored in length, width, and architecture (e.g., triplanar or biplanar) and positioned limbus-parallel or temporally to induce minimal SIA [128, 129]. Next is capsulotomy, which produces a perfectly circular, centered opening with 360-degree overlap to ensure IOL stability and reduce the risk of future tilt and decentration [130, 131]. Next, lens fragmentation involves customizable patterns that pre-soften the nucleus, decrease cumulative dissipated energy, and preserve the corneal endothelium [132].

Clinical evidence underscores the advantages of FLACS in terms of precision and safety, especially in challenging cases [133]. A meta-analysis of over 14,000 cases reports superior capsulotomy circularity and reduced phacoemulsification time, which correlates with better preservation of the corneal endothelium. For toric IOLs, FLACS-integrated digital marking may reduce misalignment, though it is not significantly better than standard phacoemulsification [134]. Limitations of FLACS include the equivocal long-term visual outcomes compared to manual techniques in uncomplicated cases, as well as anterior chamber gas bubbles that impede subsequent phacoemulsification [135].

6.2 Postoperative touch-up procedures

Despite advanced preoperative diagnostics and the integration of sophisticated IOL power calculation formulas, residual refractive errors persist in approximately 6–20% of cataract surgery cases, depending on the threshold error [1]. These discrepancies often stem from unpredictable factors, including SIA or deviations in effective lens position (ELP) due to postoperative capsular bag contraction [1, 136]. Such errors typically manifest as residual spherical or astigmatic ametropia or HOAs, which can compromise patient satisfaction. These "errors" are particularly pronounced in RCS patients, who usually have very high demands and expectations.

Touch-up procedures are generally postponed for at least 3 to 6 months after initial cataract surgery to allow for refractive stability and sufficient neuroadaptation [137]. During this time, conservative management should be prioritized to address reversible causes of dissatisfaction. This includes spectacle correction for ametropia and optimization of ocular surface disease with lubricants and anti-inflammatory agents. After careful consideration, posterior capsule opacification treatment with Nd:YAG laser can be an effective option in some cases.

Femtosecond(FS)-LASIK is the preferred touch-up method in most cases because of its rapid visual recovery, high predictability, and safety profile [138, 139]. This procedure involves creating a corneal flap with a femtosecond laser, followed by excimer laser ablation to reshape the corneal stroma bed. Wavefront-guided or topography-guided ablation profiles can further mitigate HOAs, enhancing outcomes, especially in eyes with irregular astigmatism. Studies on post-cataract LASIK demonstrate its efficacy. Uncorrected distance visual acuity (UDVA) of 20/40 or better is achieved in over 90% of patients, and refractive predictability is within ±0.50 D in over 80% [139, 140]. Detlev Breyer completely abandoned microkeratome LASIK due to its higher inherent risk of complications.

In contrast, PRK is a viable alternative for patients who are not suitable candidates for LASIK, including those with thin corneas (central thickness less than 500 μm) [141]. In PRK, the corneal epithelium is removed mechanically, with alcohol, or the excimer laser itself (transepithelially). This is followed by stromal ablation. In many cases, outcomes may are similar to LASIK for low-to-moderate corrections, although studies on post-cataract enhancement show better predictability with LASIK [142]. To counteract the subepithelial haze, mitomycin C (0.02%) is routinely applied intraoperatively [143]. However, PRK may demonstrate superiority to LASIK in cases of high myopia or irregular astigmatism. It is worth noting that PRK recovery is prolonged, involving 3 to 7 days of sometimes severe discomfort and pain, necessitating careful patient education and selection. Visual recovery may last up to 6 weeks, and corneal scarring occurs more frequently than with FS-LASIK. Therefore, FS-LASIK should be preferred in all cases, even in cases involving thin corneas or medical conditions such as Map-Dot-Fingerprint (MDF) Dystrophy.

SMILE Pro is an advanced lenticule extraction procedure based on the FS-laser technology using the VISUMAX 800 (Zeiss) [144]. It is a flapless alternative for correcting residual refractive errors in patients who have undergone cataract surgery. The procedure involves using a femtosecond laser to create an intrastromal lenticule that is then manually extracted through a small incision [145]. Although clinical evidence has proven the procedure to be an effective treatment for residual refractive errors after cataract surgery, it is limited to cases of moderate errors (−1.5 to +3.0 D) [146].

Add-on IOLs provide a reversible approach to correct residual spherical errors, because they are implanted in the ciliary sulcus, anterior to the primary IOL. Lenses such as the Sulcoflex (Rayner) and the Add-On (HumanOptics) are ideal for spherical corrections due to their simplicity and minimal invasiveness, which avoids corneal alterations [147–149]. However, toric add-on IOLs are not commonly used for astigmatism correction due to a higher risk of rotation. This risk is attributed to sulcus placement and ciliary muscle dynamics, so these lenses should be reserved for exceptional cases (off-label use).

6.3 Neuroadaptation

Neuroadaptation, the brain's capacity to reorganize visual processing pathways in response to the novel optical environment created by the implanted IOLs, is a critical and important postoperative process in RCS [53, 150]. Unlike monofocal IOLs, which provide a single clear focal point and require minimal neural adaptation, AT-IOLs distribute incoming light across multiple focal zones and often cause in initial optical artifacts, such as blurriness, halos, glare, and diminished contrast sensitivity. This process requires significant neural plasticity, whereby the visual cortex learns to prioritize relevant images while suppressing extraneous ones. This is similar to the interocular blur suppression observed in monovision corrections [151].

The timeline for neuroadaptation varies from person to person, but it generally unfolds over 3 to 6 months. Complete stabilization is possible within 12 months in some cases [150, 152]. One study examined the correlation between Mini-Mental State Examination (MMSE) completion times and adaptation speed, revealing that patients with strong baseline cognitive abilities tend to adapt more quickly following MIOL implantation [153]. Similarly, another study demonstrated that structured neuroadaptation training reduced adaptation time in MIOL recipients, highlighting the potential for targeted interventions to improve the outcomes in certain cases [154].

Despite its effectiveness for most patients, neuroadaptation sometimes fails, resulting in persistent dissatisfaction that impairs daily activities [155, 156]. The failure rate is higher with MIOLs than with EDOF IOLs because the former have a greater propensity for photopic phenomena. Important risk factors include having unrealistically high preoperative expectations and having personality traits such as perfectionism. Effective management begins clinically with thorough preoperative counseling to set realistic expectations about the adaptation period. This is the most effective strategy to mitigate these challenges. Neuroadaptation also plays a key role in stereopsis in the Duesseldorf Formula. A preoperative assessment of orthoptic status is also essential because it influences neuroadaptation and a preoperative contact lens trial may be recommended on an individual basis.

7. Conclusion

Advancements in IOL technology, preoperative diagnostics, laser-assisted surgery, personalized strategies, and touch-up procedures have transformed cataract extraction into refractive cataract surgery (RCS), which aims to correct vision and achieve spectacle independence after IOL surgery. Ophthalmologists can achieve optimal individualized outcomes by adhering to core principles, leveraging evidence-based techniques, and embracing innovations. Touch-up procedures play an essential role in RCS, as 5–20% of cases rely on them to achieve the highest degree of spectacle independence. The only disadvantage is the high cost of high-end diagnostics, continuous employee education, surgical devices, and surgeon skills. Not to mention the costs of premium ambiance and customer relations management for demanding patients.

Financial disclosure

The authors have no conflicts of interest to declare that are relevant to the content of this chapter.

A. Appendix

(See **Figures A1–A3**, Video 1, https://drive.google.com/file/d/1uDDFBeHD4mwSl4RZ9VgoCv2jxxFY6q0Z/view?usp=drive_link).

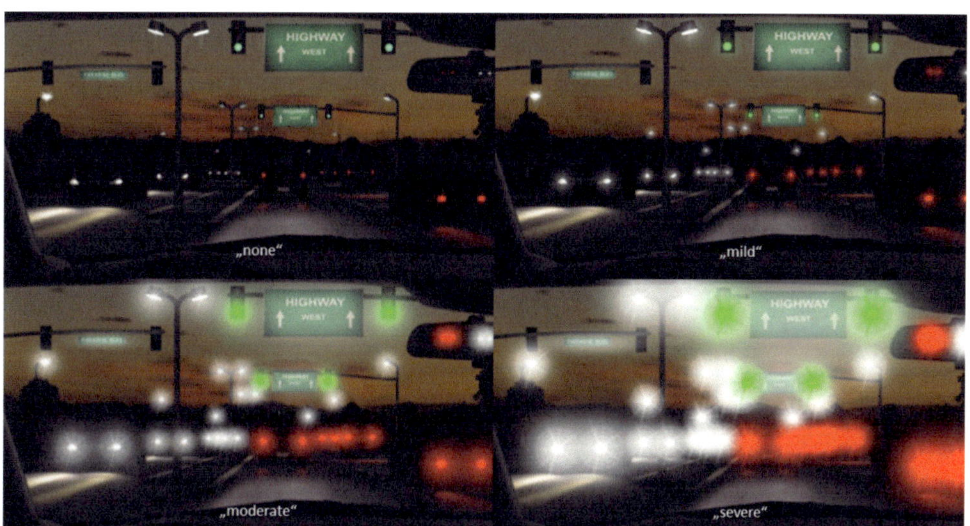

Figure A1.
Visual chart showing four different intensity levels of photopic phenomena (halos and glare) for patient counseling.

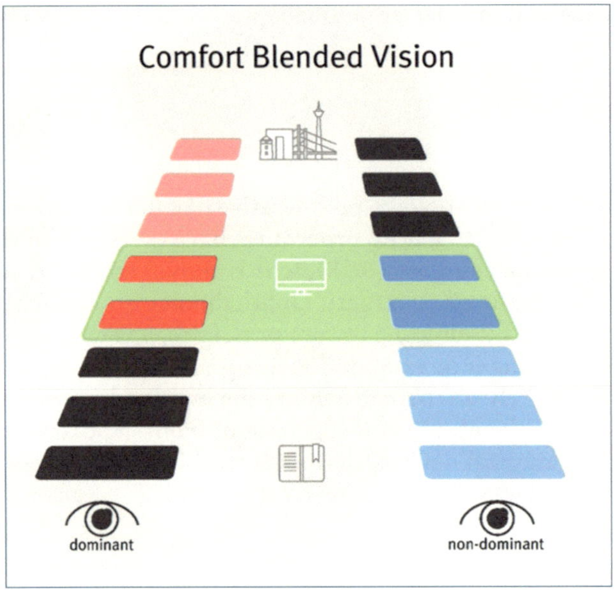

Figure A2.
Graphic illustration of "The Duesseldorf Formula", a blended vision approach.

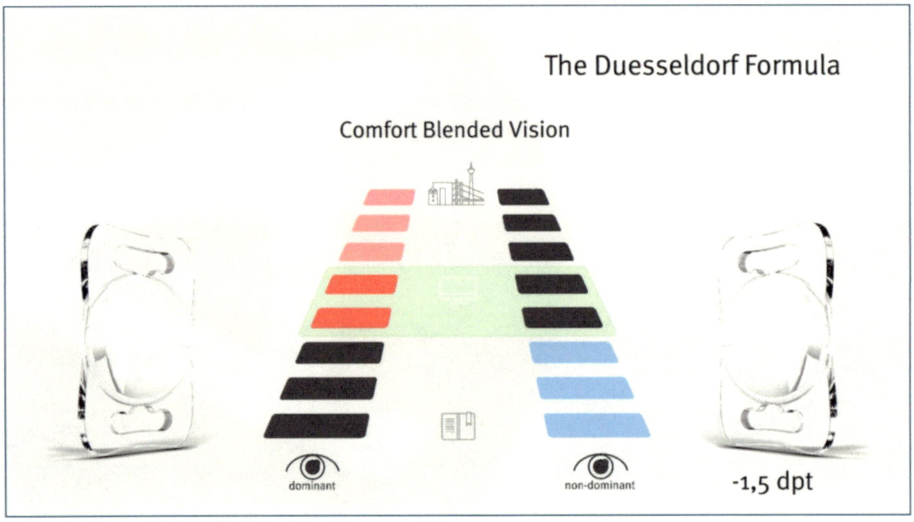

Figure A3.
Düsseldorf Formula explanation video (screenshot).

(See **Figure A4**, Video 2, https://drive.google.com/file/d/1fH0EsJpwzlj90hB1F7gta5lw7FGOAcEf/view?usp=drive_link).

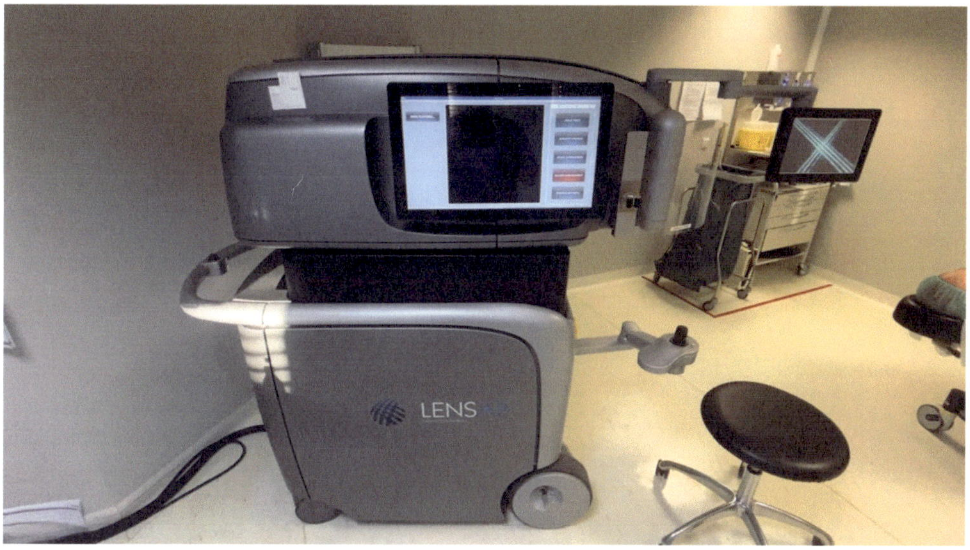

Figure A4.
LensAR femtosecond laser system.

(See **Figures A5–A13**, Video 3, https://drive.google.com/file/d/1Xf3hx5MlgsOlj3bnNEhkZhX6plDsQpWo/view?usp=drive_link).

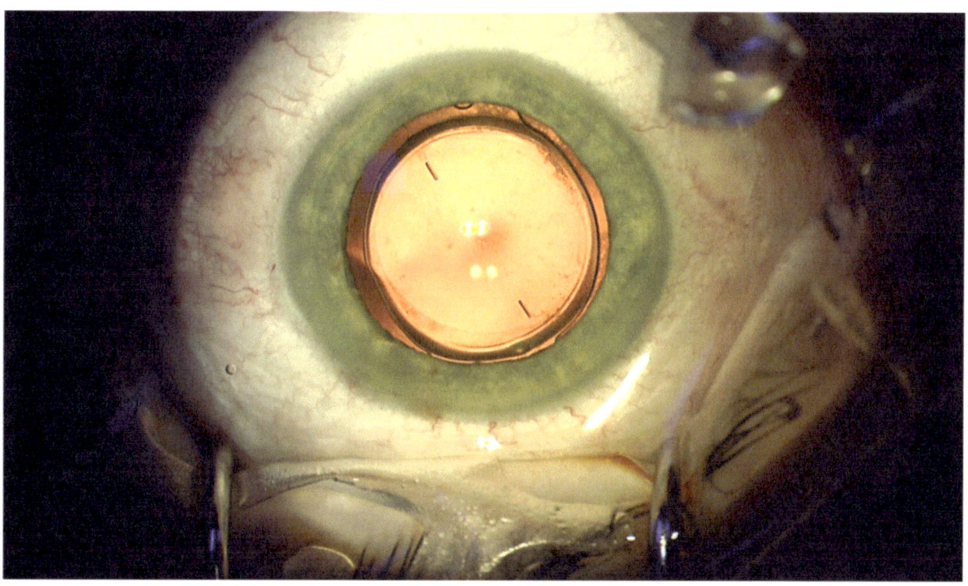

Figure A5.
Alignment of toric IOL using capsular markings in FLACS.

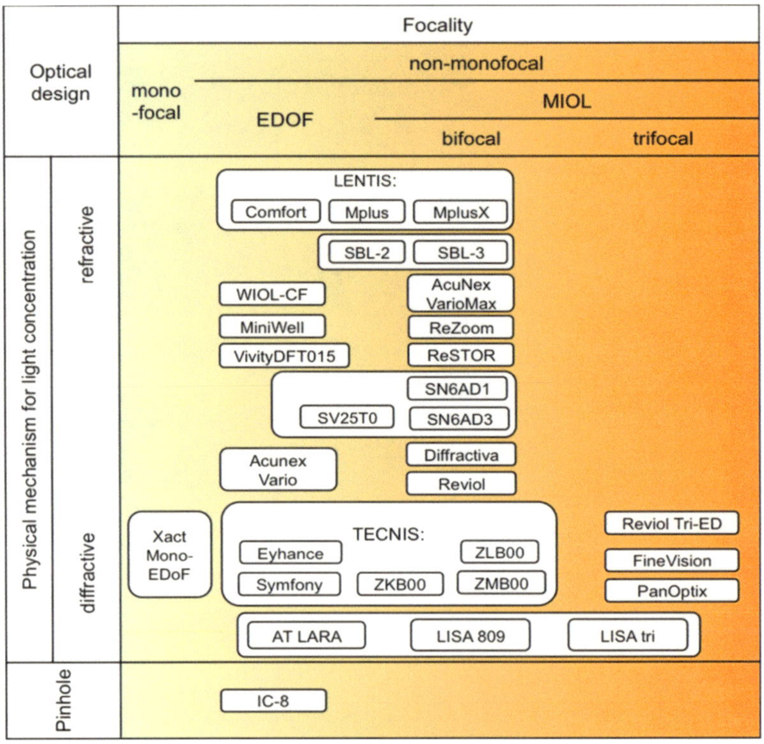

Figure A6.
A comprehensive diagram showing most of the AT-IOL currently available, categorized by focality and mechanism for light concentration.

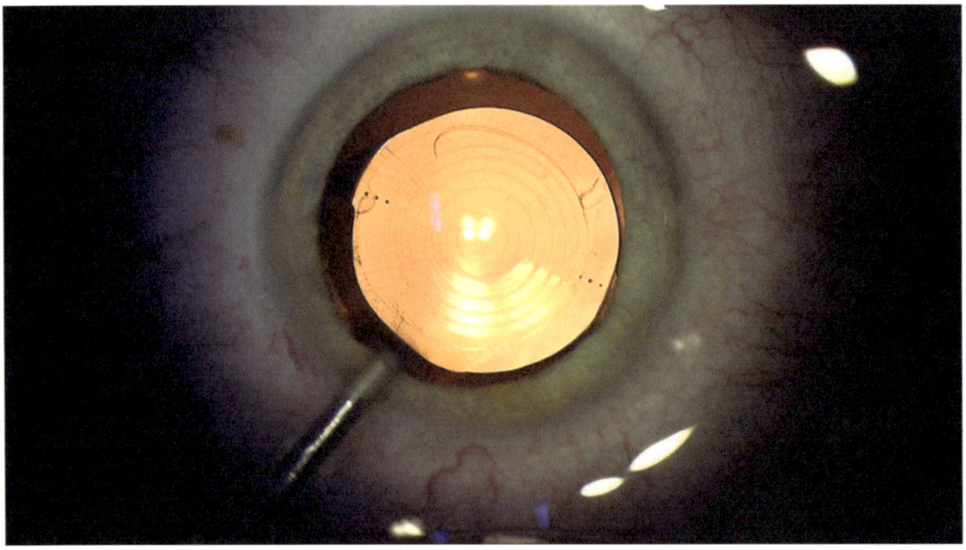

Figure A7.
Intraoperative image after PanOptix toric IOL implantation. The alignment of the IOL and FLACS markings is clearly visible.

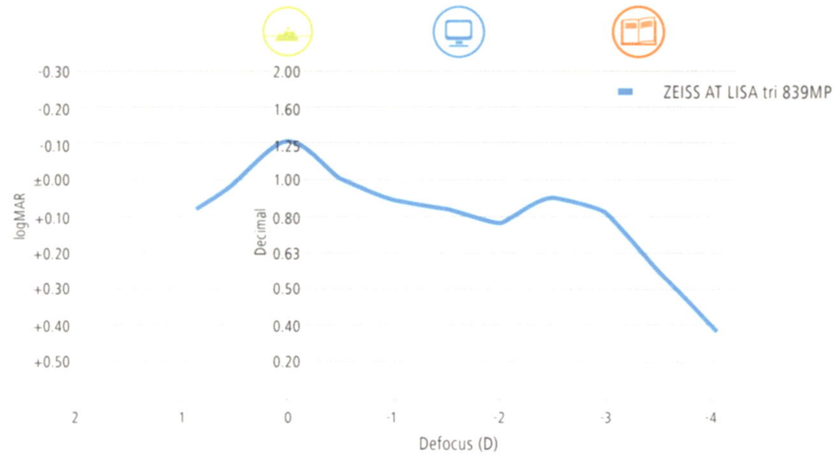

Figure A8.
Defocus curve of the LISA trifocal 839 MP [65].

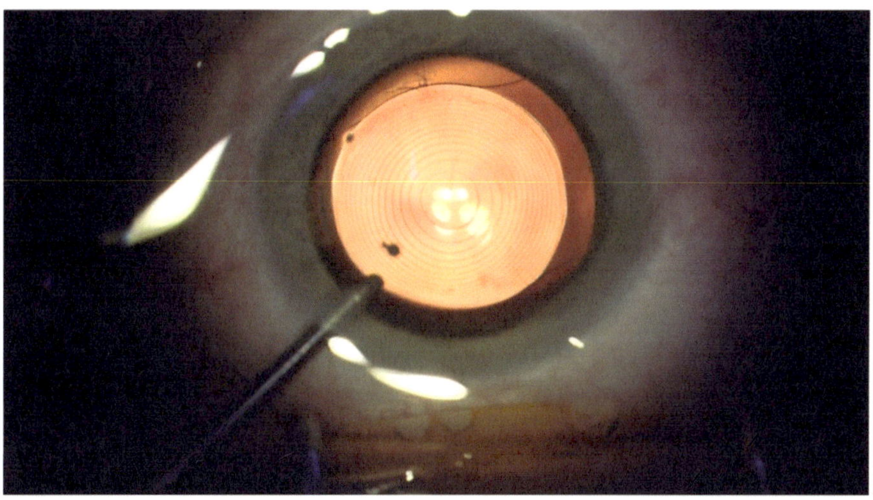

Figure A9.
Intraoperative image after LISA trifocal IOL implantation.

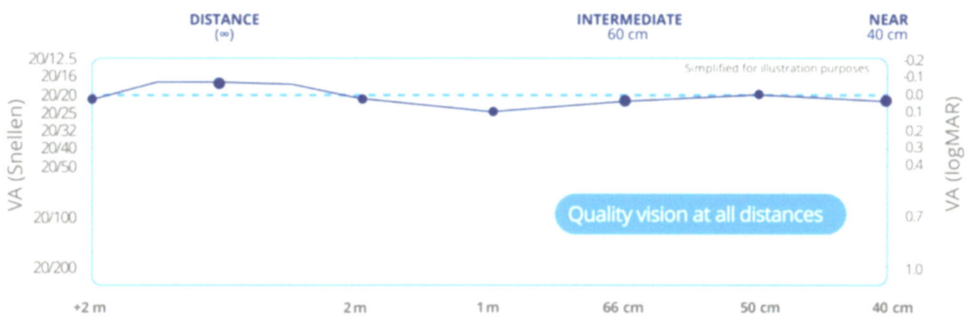

Figure A10.
Defocus curve of the PanOptix MIOL [65].

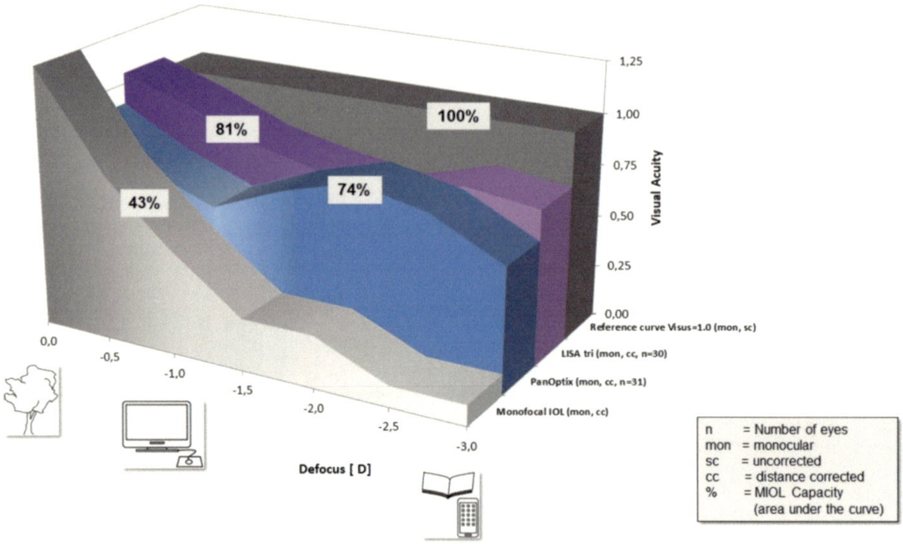

Figure A11.
Following defocus curves are presented: Reference curve (dark gray), LISA trifocal MIOL (purple), PanOptix MIOL (blue), monofocal IOL (light gray).

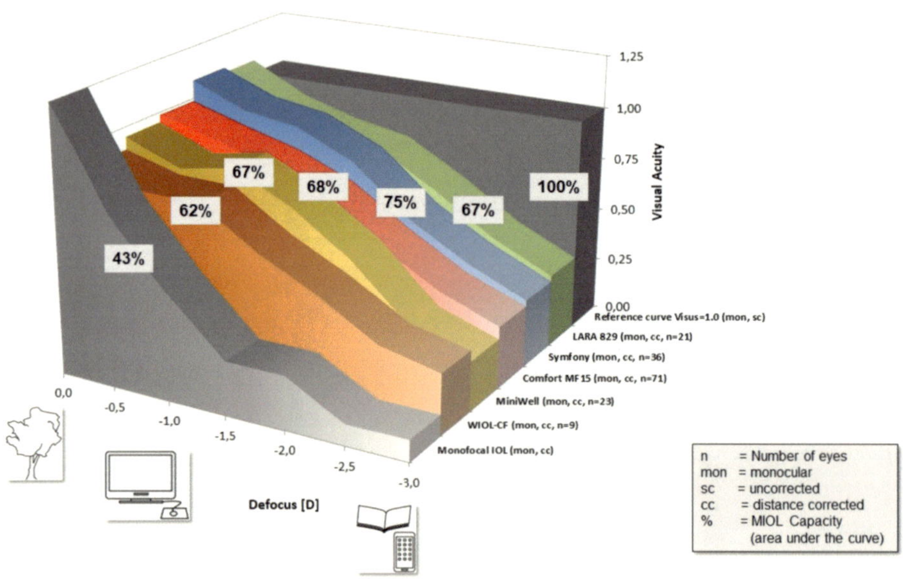

Figure A12.
Following defocus curves are presented: Reference curve (dark gray), LARA 829MP EDOF IOL (green), Tecnis Symfony EDOF IOL (blue), Lentis Comfort MF15 IOL (red), MiniWell (yellow), WIOL-CF (orange), and monofocal IOL (light grey).

DOI: http://dx.doi.org/10.5772/intechopen.1012719

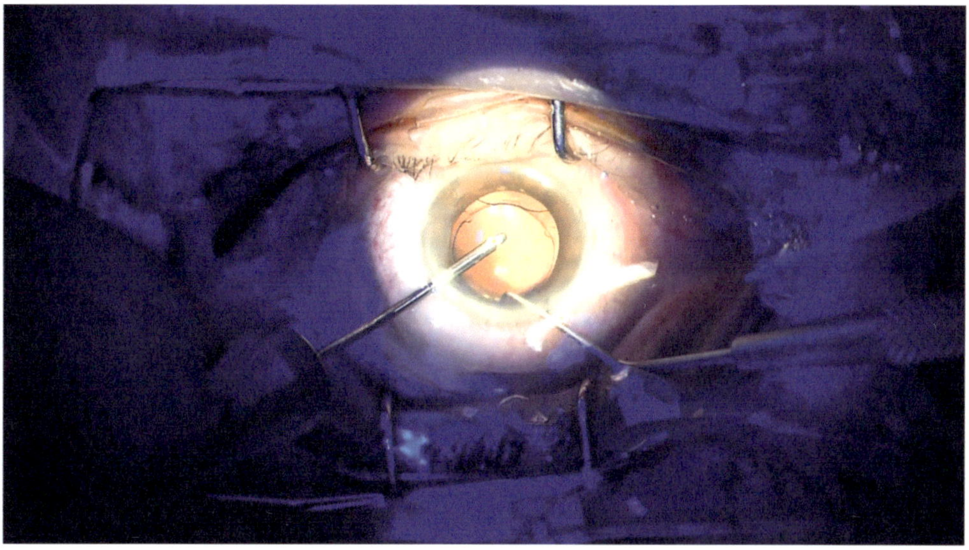

Figure A13.
Implantation of Lentis Comfort MF15 IOL.

(See **Figures A14–A22**).

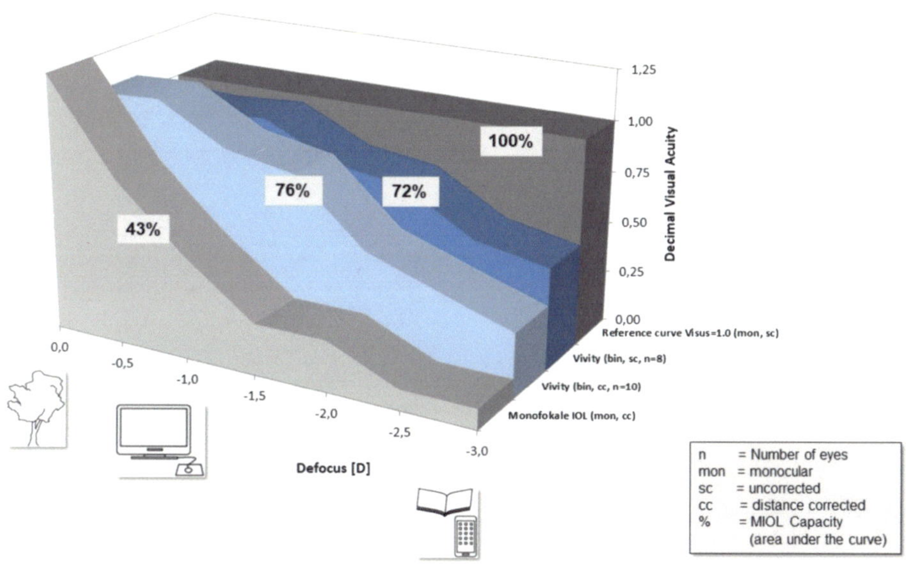

Figure A14.
Following defocus curves are presented: Reference curve (dark gray), uncorrected AcrySof IQ Vivity EDOF IOL (dark blue), corrected AcrySof IQ Vivity EDOF IOL (light blue), monofocal IOL (light gray).

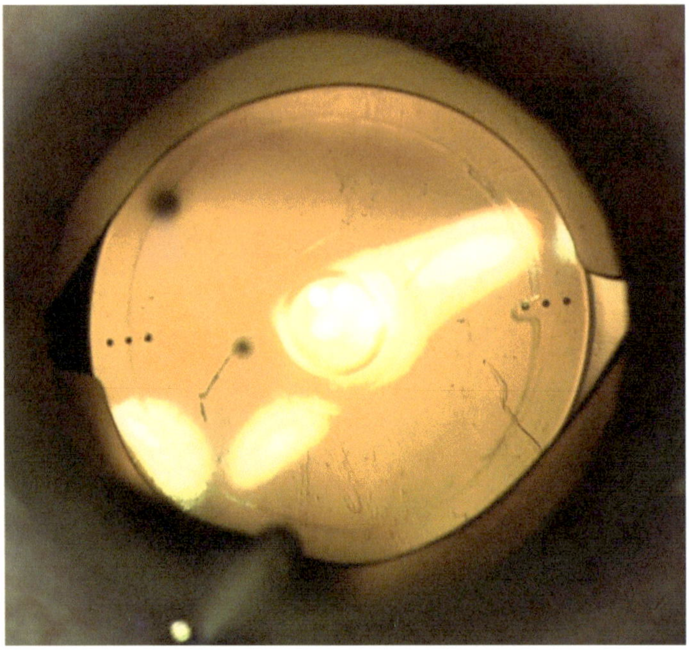

Figure A15.
Intraoperative image after Vivity EDOF toric IOL implantation. The alignment of the IOL and FLACS markings is clearly visible.

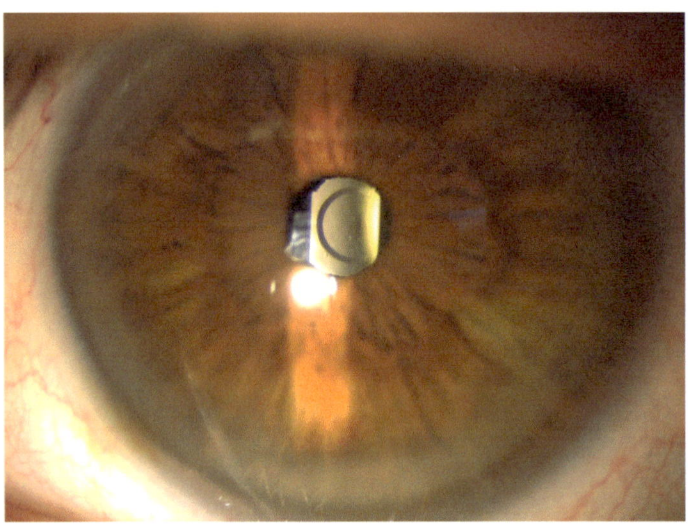

Figure A16.
Slit lamp image after Vivity EDOF toric IOL implantation.

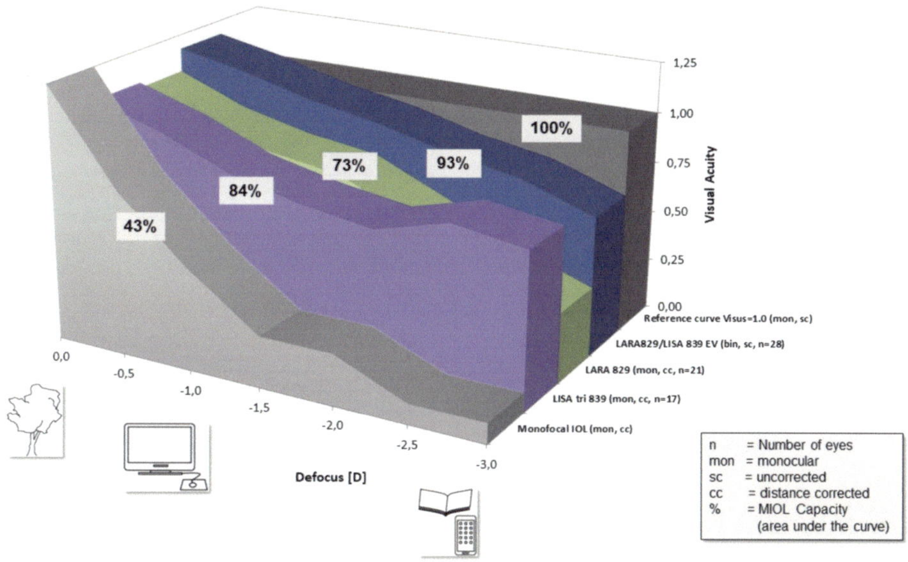

Figure A17.
Following defocus curves are presented: Reference curve (dark gray), combined LARA 829 and LISA 839 IOL (blue), LARA EDOF IOL (green), LISA trifocal MIOL (purple), monofocal IOL (light gray).

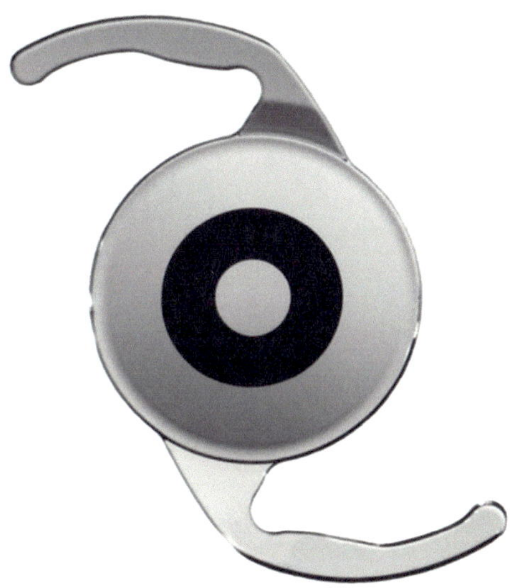

Figure A18.
The Small-Aperture IC-8 IOL [93, 94].

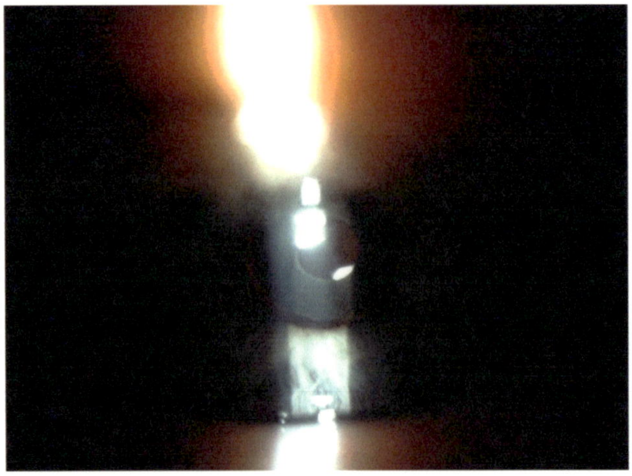

Figure A19.
Slit lamp image of the implanted IC-8 in an eye with corneal degeneration (1/2).

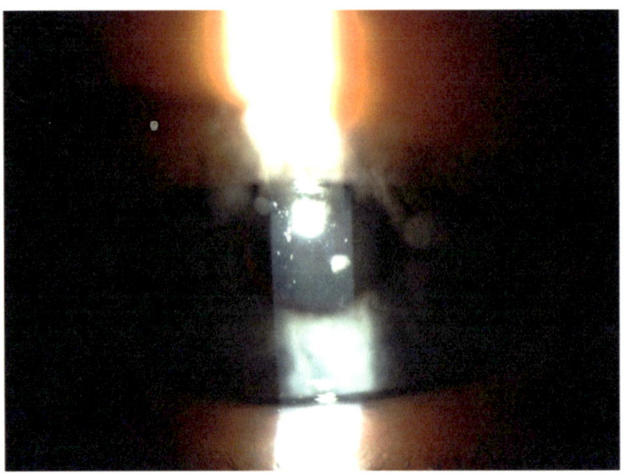

Figure A20.
Slit lamp image of the implanted IC-8 in an eye with corneal degeneration (2/2).

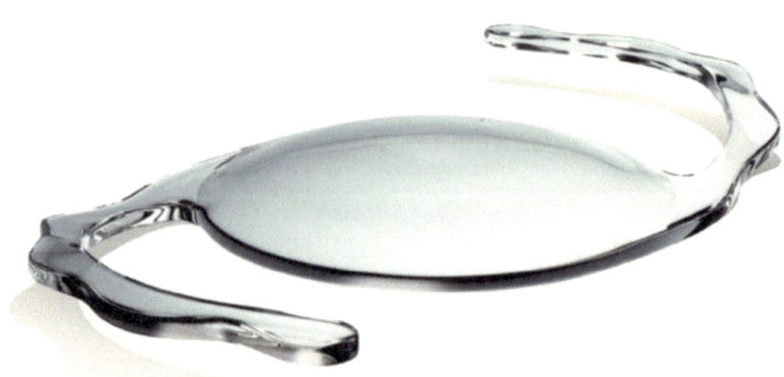

Figure A21.
The Rayner supplementary Sulcoflex aspheric IOL.

DOI: http://dx.doi.org/10.5772/intechopen.1012719

Figure A22.
A QR code providing access to lectures and in-depth resources on advanced refractive cataract surgery techniques.

Author details

Amr Saad[1,2,3,4]* and Detlev R.H. Breyer[1,2]

1 Breyer, Kaymak, Klabe Eye Surgery and Premium Eyes Düsseldorf, Germany

2 Institution for International Innovative Ophthalmic Surgery, Düsseldorf, Germany

3 Department of Ophthalmology, Stadtspital Zürich, Zurich, Switzerland

4 Spross Research Institute, Stadtspital Zürich, Zurich, Switzerland

*Address all correspondence to: a.saad@augenchirurgie.clinic

References

[1] Khoramnia R, Auffarth G, Łabuz G, Pettit G, Suryakumar R. Refractive outcomes after cataract surgery. Diagnostics (Basel). 2022;**12**(2):243. DOI: 10.3390/diagnostics12020243

[2] Narang R, Agarwal A. Refractive cataract surgery. Current Opinion in Ophthalmology. 2024;**35**(1):23-27. DOI: 10.1097/ICU.0000000000001005

[3] Donaldson K et al. Perioperative assessment for refractive cataract surgery. Journal of Cataract and Refractive Surgery. 2018;**44**(5):642-653. DOI: 10.1016/j.jcrs.2018.02.022

[4] Leffler CT, Klebanov A, Samara WA, Grzybowski A. The history of cataract surgery: From couching to phacoemulsification. Annals of Translational Medicine. 2020;**8**(22):1551. DOI: 10.21037/atm-2019-rcs-04

[5] Davis G. The evolution of cataract surgery. Missouri Medicine. 2016;**113**(1):58-62

[6] Apple DJ, Sims J. Harold Ridley and the invention of the intraocular lens. Survey of Ophthalmology. 1996;**40**(4):279-292. DOI: 10.1016/s0039-6257(96)82003-0

[7] Lim KS, Mishra A. Sir Harold Ridley as the Pioneer of intraocular lenses: His inspiration drawn from world war II pilots. Cureus. 2024;**16**(9):e68722. DOI: 10.7759/cureus.68722

[8] Gurnani B, Kaur K. Phacoemulsification. In: StatPearls. Treasure Island (FL): StatPearls Publishing; 2025. [Online]. Available from: http://www.ncbi.nlm.nih.gov/books/NBK576419/ [Accessed: July 31, 2025]

[9] Vacalebre M et al. Current state of the art and next generation of materials for a customized IntraOcular lens according to a patient-specific eye power. Polymers (Basel). 2023;**15**(6):1590. DOI: 10.3390/polym15061590

[10] Abouzeid H, Ferrini W. Femtosecond-laser assisted cataract surgery: A review. Acta Ophthalmologica. 2014;**92**(7):597-603. DOI: 10.1111/aos.12416

[11] Akella SS, Juthani VV. Extended depth of focus intraocular lenses for presbyopia. Current Opinion in Ophthalmology. 2018;**29**(4):318-322. DOI: 10.1097/ICU.0000000000000490

[12] Rampat R, Gatinel D. Multifocal and extended depth-of-focus intraocular lenses in 2020. Ophthalmology. 2021;**128**(11):e164-e185. DOI: 10.1016/j.ophtha.2020.09.026

[13] Dick HB. Accommodative intraocular lenses: current status. Current Opinion in Ophthalmology. 2005;**16**(1):8-26. DOI: 10.1097/00055735-200502000-00004

[14] Tsessler M, Cohen S, Wang L, Koch DD, Zadok D, Abulafia A. Evaluating the prediction accuracy of the hill-RBF 3.0 formula using a heteroscedastic statistical method. Journal of Cataract and Refractive Surgery. 2022;**48**(1):37-43. DOI: 10.1097/j.jcrs.0000000000000702

[15] Debellemanière G et al. The PEARL-DGS formula: The development of an open-source machine learning-based thick IOL calculation formula. American Journal of Ophthalmology. 2021;**232**:58-69. DOI: 10.1016/j.ajo.2021.05.004

[16] Chang DF et al. ASCRS white paper: Clinical review of intraoperative floppy-iris syndrome. Journal of Cataract and Refractive Surgery. 2008;**34**(12):2153-2162. DOI: 10.1016/j.jcrs.2008.08.031

[17] Manoharan N et al. Refractive outcomes of phacoemulsification cataract surgery in glaucoma patients. Journal of Cataract and Refractive Surgery. 2018;**44**(3):348-354. DOI: 10.1016/j.jcrs.2017.12.024

[18] Nicholson M et al. Current concepts in the management of cataract with keratoconus. Indian Journal of Ophthalmology. 2024;**72**(4):508-519. DOI: 10.4103/IJO.IJO_1241_23

[19] Biscevic A, Ahmedbegovic-Pjano M, Pasalic A, Ziga N, Gabric K, Bohac M. Changes in the higher order ocular aberrations and central corneal thickness after T-PRK and fs-LASIK. Acta Informatica Medica. 2020;**28**(2):98-102. DOI: 10.5455/aim.2020.28.98-102

[20] Wielders LHP et al. Prevention of cystoid macular Edema after cataract surgery in nondiabetic and diabetic patients: A systematic review and meta-analysis. American Journal of Ophthalmology. 2015;**160**(5):968-981.e33. DOI: 10.1016/j.ajo.2015.07.032

[21] Höhn F et al. Functional results one year after implantation of a Bitoric, trifocal intraocular lens. Klinische Monatsblätter für Augenheilkunde. 2015;**232**(8):957-961. DOI: 10.1055/s-0041-103335

[22] Pedrotti E et al. Comparative analysis of visual outcomes with 4 intraocular lenses: Monofocal, multifocal, and extended range of vision. Journal of Cataract and Refractive Surgery. 2018;**44**(2):156-167. DOI: 10.1016/j.jcrs.2017.11.011

[23] Tchah H, Nam K, Yoo A. Predictive factors for photic phenomena after refractive, rotationally asymmetric, multifocal intraocular lens implantation. International Journal of Ophthalmology. 2017;**10**(2):241-245. DOI: 10.18240/ijo.2017.02.10

[24] Saad A, Frings A, Druchkiv V, Katz T. Pre- and postoperative angle kappa in MIOL patients after touch-up LASIK. PLoS One. 2023;**18**(4):e0283578. DOI: 10.1371/journal.pone.0283578

[25] Fernández J, Ribeiro F, Burguera N, Burguera-Giménez N, Rodríguez-Vallejo M. Replacing theories with evidence around the axes of the eye in intraocular lens selection: A review for the clinician. Ophthalmology and Therapy. 2025;**14**(3):471-487. DOI: 10.1007/s40123-025-01092-4

[26] Pepose JS et al. Assessing ocular dominance: Rethinking the current paradigm. Journal of Cataract and Refractive Surgery. 2025;**51**(7):592-599. DOI: 10.1097/j.jcrs.0000000000001659

[27] Sheppard JD, Nichols KK. Dry eye disease associated with Meibomian gland dysfunction: Focus on tear film characteristics and the therapeutic landscape. Ophthalmology and Therapy. 2023;**12**(3):1397-1418. DOI: 10.1007/s40123-023-00669-1

[28] Chung HS, Rhim JW, Park JH. Combination treatment with intense pulsed light, thermal pulsation (LipiFlow), and meibomian gland expression for refractory meibomian gland dysfunction. International Ophthalmology. 2022;**42**(11):3311-3319. DOI: 10.1007/s10792-022-02330-5

[29] Goudie C, Tatham A, Davies R, Sifton A, Wright M. The effect of the timing of the cessation of contact lens

use on the results of biometry. Eye (London, England). 2018;**32**(6):1048-1054. DOI: 10.1038/s41433-018-0019-1

[30] Santhiago MR et al. Association between the percent tissue altered and post-laser in situ keratomileusis ectasia in eyes with normal preoperative topography. American Journal of Ophthalmology. 2014;**158**(1):87-95.e1. DOI: 10.1016/j.ajo.2014.04.002

[31] Yang C, An Q, Zhou H, Ge H. Research progress on the impact of cataract surgery on corneal endothelial cells. Advances in Ophthalmology Practice and Research. 2024;**4**(4):194-201. DOI: 10.1016/j.aopr.2024.08.002

[32] Daien V, Le Pape A, Heve D, Carriere I, Villain M. Incidence, risk factors, and impact of age on retinal detachment after cataract surgery in France: A National Population Study. Ophthalmology. 2015;**122**(11):2179-2185. DOI: 10.1016/j.ophtha.2015.07.014

[33] Rudalevicius P, Lekaviciene R, Auffarth GU, Liutkeviciene R, Jasinskas V. Relations between patient personality and patients‘ dissatisfaction after multifocal intraocular lens implantation: Clinical study based on the five factor inventory personality evaluation. Eye (London, England). 2020;**34**(4):717-724. DOI: 10.1038/s41433-019-0585-x

[34] Baenninger PB, Faes L, Kaufmann C, Reichmuth V, Bachmann LM, Thiel MA. Efficiency of video-presented information about excimer laser treatment on ametropic patients' knowledge and satisfaction with the informed consent process. Journal of Cataract and Refractive Surgery. 2018;**44**(12):1426-1430. DOI: 10.1016/j.jcrs.2018.07.052

[35] Newman-Casey PA et al. The effect of Counseling on cataract patient knowledge, decisional conflict, and satisfaction. Ophthalmic Epidemiology. 2015;**22**(6):387-393. DOI: 10.3109/09286586.2015.1066016

[36] Dai J et al. Current status of shared decision-making in intraocular lens selection for cataract surgery: A cross-sectional study. Patient Preference and Adherence. 2024;**18**:1311-1321. DOI: 10.2147/PPA.S468452

[37] Marcos S, Artal P, Lundström L, Yoon G. Visual simulation of intraocular lenses: Technologies and applications [invited]. Biomedical Optics Express. 2025;**16**(3):1025-1042. DOI: 10.1364/BOE.546971

[38] Salerno LC, Tiveron MC, Alió JL. Multifocal intraocular lenses: Types, outcomes, complications and how to solve them. Taiwan Journal of Ophthalmology. 2017;7(4):179-184. DOI: 10.4103/tjo.tjo_19_17

[39] Breyer DRH, Kaymak H, Ax T, Kretz FTA, Auffarth GU, Hagen PR. Multifocal intraocular lenses and extended depth of focus intraocular lenses. Asia-Pacific Journal of Ophthalmology (Phila). 2017;**6**(4):339-349. DOI: 10.22608/APO.2017186

[40] Auffarth G, Rabsilber T, Kohnen T, Holzer M. Design and optical principles of multifocal lenses. Der Ophthalmologe : Zeitschrift der Deutschen Ophthalmologischen Gesellschaft. 2008;**105**:522-526

[41] Duffey RJ, Zabel RW, Lindstrom RL. Multifocal intraocular lenses. Journal of Cataract and Refractive Surgery. 1990;**16**(4):423-429. DOI: 10.1016/s0886-3350(13)80794-8

[42] Simpson MJ et al. Design concepts for advanced-technology intraocular lenses [invited]. Biomedical Optics

Express. 2024;**16**(1):334-361. DOI: 10.1364/BOE.544647

[43] Bellucci R. Multifocal intraocular lenses. Current Opinion in Ophthalmology. 2005;**16**:33-37. DOI: 10.1097/00055735-200502000-00006

[44] Alio JL, Plaza-Puche AB, Férnandez-Buenaga R, Pikkel J, Maldonado M. Multifocal intraocular lenses: An overview. Survey of Ophthalmology. 2017;**62**(5):611-634. DOI: 10.1016/j.survophthal.2017.03.005

[45] Sudhir RR, Dey A, Bhattacharrya S, Bahulayan A. AcrySof IQ PanOptix intraocular lens versus extended depth of focus intraocular lens and trifocal intraocular lens: A clinical overview. Asia-Pacific Journal of Ophthalmology (Phila). 2019;**8**(4):335-349. DOI: 10.1097/APO.0000000000000253

[46] Zelichowska B, Rekas M, Stankiewicz A, Cerviño A, Montés-Micó R. Apodized diffractive versus refractive multifocal intraocular lenses: Optical and visual evaluation. Journal of Cataract & Refractive Surgery. 2008;**34**(12):2036. DOI: 10.1016/j.jcrs.2008.06.045

[47] Kohnen T et al. Visual outcomes after implantation of a segmental refractive multifocal intraocular lens following cataract surgery. American Journal of Ophthalmology. 2018;**191**:156-165. DOI: 10.1016/j.ajo.2018.04.011

[48] Dick HB et al. Comparison of 3-month visual outcomes of a new multifocal intraocular lens vs a trifocal intraocular lens. Journal of Cataract and Refractive Surgery. 2022;**48**(11):1270-1276. DOI: 10.1097/j.jcrs.0000000000000971

[49] Łabuz G, Yan W, Baur ID, Khoramnia R, Auffarth GU. Comparison of five presbyopia-correcting intraocular lenses: Optical-bench assessment with visual-quality simulation. Journal of Clinical Medicine. Jan 2023;**12**(7):2523. DOI: 10.3390/jcm12072523

[50] Cho J-Y et al. Visual outcomes and optical quality of accommodative, multifocal, extended depth-of-focus, and Monofocal intraocular lenses in presbyopia-correcting cataract surgery: A systematic review and Bayesian network meta-analysis. JAMA Ophthalmology. Nov 2022;**140**(11):1045-1053. DOI: 10.1001/jamaophthalmol.2022.3667

[51] Zhang Z, Jiang H, Zhou H, Zhou F. Comparative efficacy between trifocal and bifocal intraocular lens among patients undergoing cataract surgery: A systematic review and meta-analysis. Frontiers in Medicine (Lausanne). 2021;**8**:647268. DOI: 10.3389/fmed.2021.647268

[52] Xu X, Zhu M-M, Zou H-D. Refractive versus diffractive multifocal intraocular lenses in cataract surgery: A meta-analysis of randomized controlled trials. Journal of Refractive Surgery. 2014;**30**(9):634-644. DOI: 10.3928/1081597X-20140814-04

[53] Rosa AM et al. Functional magnetic resonance imaging to assess neuroadaptation to multifocal intraocular lenses. Journal of Cataract and Refractive Surgery. 2017;**43**(10):1287-1296. DOI: 10.1016/j.jcrs.2017.07.031

[54] Chang JSM, Ng JCM, Chan VKC, Law AKP. Visual outcomes and patient satisfaction after refractive lens exchange with a single-piece diffractive multifocal intraocular lens. Journal of Ophthalmology. 2014;**2014**:458296. DOI: 10.1155/2014/458296

[55] Nuzzi R, Tripoli F, Ghilardi A. Evaluation of the effects of multifocal

intraocular lens Oculentis LENTIS Mplus LS-313 MF30 on visual performance in patients affected by bilateral cataract and treated with phacoemulsification. Journal of Ophthalmology. 2022;**2022**:1315480. DOI: 10.1155/2022/1315480

[56] Venter JA, Pelouskova M, Collins BM, Schallhorn SC, Hannan SJ. Visual outcomes and patient satisfaction in 9366 eyes using a refractive segmented multifocal intraocular lens. Journal of Cataract and Refractive Surgery. 2013;**39**(10):1477-1484. DOI: 10.1016/j.jcrs.2013.03.035

[57] Kawamura J, Tanabe H, Shojo T, Yamauchi T, Takase K, Tabuchi H. Comparison of visual performance between diffractive bifocal and diffractive trifocal intraocular lenses. Scientific Reports. 2024;**14**(1):5292. DOI: 10.1038/s41598-024-55926-5

[58] Tanabe H, Shojo T, Yamauchi T, Takase K, Akada M, Tabuchi H. Comparative visual performance of diffractive bifocal and rotationally asymmetric refractive intraocular lenses. Scientific Reports. 2022;**12**(1):19394. DOI: 10.1038/s41598-022-24123-7

[59] Ravalico G, Baccara F, Rinaldi G. Contrast sensitivity in multifocal intraocular lenses. Journal of Cataract & Refractive Surgery. 1993;**19**(1):22. DOI: 10.1016/S0886-3350(13)80274-X

[60] Schmickler S, Bautista CP, Goes F, Shah S, Wolffsohn JS. Clinical evaluation of a multifocal aspheric diffractive intraocular lens. The British Journal of Ophthalmology. 2013;**97**(12):1560-1564. DOI: 10.1136/bjophthalmol-2013-304010

[61] Lubiński W, Gronkowska-Serafin J, Podborączyńska-Jodko K. Clinical outcomes after cataract surgery with implantation of the Tecnis ZMB00 multifocal intraocular lens. Medical Science Monitor. 2014;**20**:1220-1226. DOI: 10.12659/MSM.890585

[62] Ye L, Chen T, Hu Z, Yang Q, Su Q, Li J. Comparison of the visual performance between oculentis MF30 and Tecnis ZMB00 multifocal intraocular lenses. Annals of Translational Medicine. 2021;**9**(2):144. DOI: 10.21037/atm-20-7777

[63] Yoon CH, Shin I-S, Kim MK. Trifocal versus bifocal diffractive intraocular lens implantation after cataract surgery or refractive lens exchange: A meta-analysis. Journal of Korean Medical Science. 2018;**33**(44):e275. DOI: 10.3346/jkms.2018.33.e275

[64] Ison M, Scott J, Apel J, Apel A. Patient expectation, satisfaction and clinical outcomes with a new multifocal intraocular lens. Clinical Ophthalmology. 2021;**15**:4131-4140. DOI: 10.2147/OPTH.S327424

[65] Böhm M, Hemkeppler E, Kohnen T. Self-rated quality of vision and optical phenomena intensity of diffractive presbyopia-correcting IOLs: EDoF, trifocal vs panfocal. Journal of Cataract and Refractive Surgery. 2022;**48**(8):877-886. DOI: 10.1097/j.jcrs.0000000000000862

[66] Xu Z, Cao D, Chen X, Wu S, Wang X, Wu Q. Comparison of clinical performance between trifocal and bifocal intraocular lenses: A meta-analysis. PLoS One. 2017;**12**(10):e0186522. DOI: 10.1371/journal.pone.0186522

[67] Law EM, Aggarwal RK, Kasaby H. Clinical outcomes with a new trifocal intraocular lens. European Journal of Ophthalmology. 2014;**24**(4):501-508. DOI: 10.5301/ejo.5000407

[68] Ribeiro FJ, Ferreira TB, Silva D, Matos AC, Gaspar S. Visual outcomes

and patient satisfaction after implantation of a presbyopia-correcting intraocular lens that combines extended depth-of-focus and multifocal profiles. Journal of Cataract and Refractive Surgery. 2021;**47**(11):1448-1453. DOI: 10.1097/j.jcrs.0000000000000659

[69] De Rojas JO, Sandoval HP, Potvin R, Solomon KD. Visual outcomes, quality of vision, patient satisfaction and spectacle Independence after bilateral implantation of the synergy™ intraocular lens. Clinical Ophthalmology. 2023;**17**:2277-2285. DOI: 10.2147/OPTH.S421185

[70] Gabrić N, Gabrić I, Gabrić K, Biščević A, Piñero DP, Bohač M. Clinical outcomes with a new continuous range of vision presbyopia-correcting intraocular lens. Journal of Refractive Surgery. 2021;**37**(4):256-262. DOI: 10.3928/1081597X-20210209-01

[71] Kanclerz P, Toto F, Grzybowski A, Alio JL. Extended depth-of-field intraocular lenses: An update. Asia-Pacific Journal of Ophthalmology (Phila). 2020;**9**(3):194-202. DOI: 10.1097/APO.0000000000000296

[72] Megiddo-Barnir E, Alió JL. Latest development in extended depth-of-focus intraocular lenses: An update. Asia-Pacific Journal of Ophthalmology (Phila). 2023;**12**(1):58-79. DOI: 10.1097/APO.0000000000000590

[73] Kohnen T et al. Visual performance of an extended depth of focus intraocular lens for treatment selection. Eye (London, England). 2019;**33**(10):1556-1563. DOI: 10.1038/s41433-019-0443-x

[74] Tañá-Sanz S, Tañá-Sanz P, Elvira-Giner B, Orts-Vila P, Tañá-Rivero P. Visual performance, light distortion and patient reported outcomes with a new bi-aspheric non-diffractive extended depth of focus intraocular lens. Frontiers in Medicine (Lausanne). 2025;**12**:1513803. DOI: 10.3389/fmed.2025.1513803

[75] Baur ID, Yan W, Auffarth GU, Khoramnia R, Łabuz G. Optical quality and higher order aberrations of refractive extended depth of focus intraocular lenses. Journal of Refractive Surgery. 2023;**39**(10):668-674. DOI: 10.3928/1081597X-20230831-01

[76] Baur ID, Auffarth GU, Yan W, Łabuz G, Khoramnia R. Visualization of ray propagation through extended depth-of-focus intraocular lenses. Diagnostics (Basel). 2022;**12**(11):2667. DOI: 10.3390/diagnostics12112667

[77] Schmid R, Borkenstein AF. Enhanced depth of focus intraocular lenses: Through focus evaluation of Wavefront-shaping versus diffractive optics. Biomedicine Hub. 2023;**8**(1):25-30. DOI: 10.1159/000529234

[78] Ang RET, Araneta MMQ, Cruz EM. Review of surgical devices using small aperture optics. Taiwan Journal of Ophthalmology. 2022;**12**(3):282-294. DOI: 10.4103/tjo.tjo_45_21

[79] Kohnen T et al. Nondiffractive wavefront-shaping extended depth-of-focus intraocular lens: Visual performance and patient-reported outcomes. Journal of Cataract and Refractive Surgery. 2022;**48**(2):144-150. DOI: 10.1097/j.jcrs.0000000000000826

[80] Sánchez-González J-M, Sánchez-González MC, De-Hita-Cantalejo C, Ballesteros-Sánchez A. Small aperture IC-8 extended-depth-of-focus intraocular lens in cataract surgery: A systematic review. Journal of Clinical Medicine. Jan 2022;**11**(16):4654. DOI: 10.3390/jcm11164654

[81] Packer M, Monteiro T, Schweitzer C, Rosen P. Prospective, randomized, controlled multicenter study of a monofocal extended depth of focus IOL compared to a standard aspheric monofocal IOL. Journal of Cataract and Refractive Surgery. 2025. DOI: 10.1097/j.jcrs.0000000000001672

[82] Corbett D et al. Quality of vision clinical outcomes for a new fully-refractive extended depth of focus intraocular lens. Eye. 2024;**38**(1):9-14. DOI: 10.1038/s41433-024-03039-8

[83] Rodov L, Reitblat O, Levy A, Assia EI, Kleinmann G. Visual outcomes and patient satisfaction for trifocal, extended depth of focus and monofocal intraocular lenses. Journal of Refractive Surgery. 2019;**35**(7):434-440. DOI: 10.3928/1081597X-20190618-01

[84] Oshika T et al. One-year clinical evaluation of rotationally asymmetric multifocal intraocular lens with +1.5 diopters near addition. Scientific Reports. 2019;**9**:13117. DOI: 10.1038/s41598-019-49524-z

[85] Pedrotti E et al. Quality of vision, patient satisfaction and long-term visual function after bilateral implantation of a low addition multifocal intraocular lens. International Ophthalmology. 2018;**38**(4):1709-1716. DOI: 10.1007/s10792-017-0652-x

[86] Nakajima D, Takahashi H, Kobayakawa S. Clinical outcome of Lentis comfort intraocular lens implantation. Journal of Nippon Medical School. 2021;**88**(5):398-407. DOI: 10.1272/jnms.JNMS.2021_88-504

[87] Campos N et al. Preliminary clinical outcomes of a new enhanced depth of focus intraocular lens. Clinical Ophthalmology. 2021;**15**:4801-4807. DOI: 10.2147/OPTH.S344379

[88] Campos N. Clinical outcomes and patient satisfaction of an enhanced depth of focus intraocular lens targeted for mini-monovision. Clinical Ophthalmology. 2024;**18**:1607-1613. DOI: 10.2147/OPTH.S459868

[89] Cochener B, C. S. Group. Clinical outcomes of a new extended range of vision intraocular lens: International Multicenter Concerto Study. Journal of Cataract & Refractive Surgery. 2016;**42**(9):1268. DOI: 10.1016/j.jcrs.2016.06.033

[90] Chang DH et al. Visual outcomes and safety of an extended depth-of-focus intraocular lens: Results of a pivotal clinical trial. Journal of Cataract & Refractive Surgery. 2022;**48**(3):288. DOI: 10.1097/j.jcrs.0000000000000747

[91] Tavassoli S et al. Trifocal versus extended depth of focus (EDOF) intraocular lenses after cataract extraction. Cochrane Database of Systematic Reviews. 2024;**7**(7):CD014891. DOI: 10.1002/14651858.CD014891.pub2

[92] Reinhard T et al. Comparison of two extended depth of focus intraocular lenses with a monofocal lens: A multi-centre randomised trial. Graefe's Archive for Clinical and Experimental Ophthalmology. 2021;**259**(2):431-442. DOI: 10.1007/s00417-020-04868-5

[93] McCabe C et al. Clinical outcomes in a U.S. registration study of a new EDOF intraocular lens with a nondiffractive design. Journal of Cataract and Refractive Surgery. 2022;**48**(11):1297-1304. DOI: 10.1097/j.jcrs.0000000000000978

[94] Howes F et al. Visual performance and patient satisfaction of bilaterally implanted extended depth of focus intraocular lens: Outcomes of a

multicenter registry. Journal of Refractive Surgery. 2025;**41**(2):e131-e143. DOI: 10.3928/1081597X-20241230-01

[95] Hovanesian JA, Jones M, Allen Q. The vivity extended range of vision IOL vs the PanOptix trifocal, ReStor 2.5 active focus and ReStor 3.0 multifocal lenses: A comparison of patient satisfaction, visual disturbances, and spectacle Independence. Clinical Ophthalmology. Jan 2022;**16**:145-152. DOI: 10.2147/OPTH.S347382

[96] Vukich J, Modi S, Fisher BL, Stonecipher K, Lin L, Michna M. Clinical comparison of a small-aperture intraocular lens versus a monofocal control. Journal of Refractive Surgery. 2024;**40**(11):e824-e835. DOI: 10.3928/1081597X-20240731-02

[97] Breyer DR, Lücht D, Kirca M, Beckers L, Kretz F, Auffarth G. Evaluation of the Quality of Visual Acuity, Stereoacuity, and Photic Phenomena after Bilateral Implantation of a Rotational Asymmetric Enhanced Depth of Focus Intraocular Lens in a Blended Vision Strategy. 2023

[98] Solomon KD, Sandoval HP, Potvin R. Visual outcomes, satisfaction, and spectacle independence with a nondiffractive extended vision intraocular lens targeted for slight monovision. Journal of Cataract and Refractive Surgery. 2023;**49**(7):686-690. DOI: 10.1097/j.jcrs.0000000000001191

[99] Levy I, Shah RP, Mukhija R, Nanavaty MA. Outcomes of mini-monovision with monofocal, enhanced monofocal and extended depth-of-focus intraocular lenses. Frontiers in Medicine (Lausanne). 2025;**12**:1522383. DOI: 10.3389/fmed.2025.1522383

[100] Fernández J, Rocha-de-Lossada C, Zamorano-Martín F, Rodríguez-Calvo-de-Mora M, Rodríguez-Vallejo M. Positioning of enhanced monofocal intraocular lenses between conventional monofocal and extended depth of focus lenses: A scoping review. BMC Ophthalmology. 2023;**23**:101. DOI: 10.1186/s12886-023-02844-1

[101] Vega F, Millán MS, Gil MA, Garzón N. Optical performance of a Monofocal intraocular lens designed to extend depth of focus. Journal of Refractive Surgery. 2020;**36**(9):625-632. DOI: 10.3928/1081597X-20200710-01

[102] Alarcon A, Cánovas C, Koopman B, Weeber H, Auffarth GU, Piers PA. Enhancing the intermediate vision of Monofocal intraocular lenses using a higher order aspheric optic. Journal of Refractive Surgery. 2020;**36**(8):520-527. DOI: 10.3928/1081597X-20200612-01

[103] Goslings O, Veraart H, van de Laar-Muskens J, Piñero DP. Clinical outcomes with an aspheric monofocal and a new enhanced monofocal intraocular lens with modified optical profile. Graefe's Archive for Clinical and Experimental Ophthalmology. 2023;**261**(8):2315-2326. DOI: 10.1007/s00417-023-06128-8

[104] Łabuz G, Son H-S, Naujokaitis T, Yildirim TM, Khoramnia R, Auffarth GU. Laboratory investigation of preclinical visual-quality metrics and halo-size in enhanced monofocal intraocular lenses. Ophthalmology and Therapy. 2021;**10**(4):1093-1104. DOI: 10.1007/s40123-021-00411-9

[105] Alarcon A, Canovas C, Koopman B, Pande MV, Koch DD, Piers P. Optical bench evaluation of the effect of pupil size in new generation monofocal intraocular lenses. BMC Ophthalmology. 2023;**23**(1):112. DOI: 10.1186/s12886-023-02839-y

[106] García-Bella J, Burgos-Blasco B, Vidal-Villegas B, Garzón N, Villanueva C,

García-Feijoo J. Visual and refractive outcomes after bilateral implantation of an enhanced monofocal intraocular lens: Prospective study. Journal of Cataract and Refractive Surgery. 2024;**50**(6):585-590. DOI: 10.1097/j.jcrs.0000000000001422

[107] Miret JJ, Camps VJ, García C, Caballero MT, Gonzalez-Leal JM. Analysis of the optical performance of intraocular lenses using profilometric measurements. Graefe's Archive for Clinical and Experimental Ophthalmology. 2025;**263**(2):451-465. DOI: 10.1007/s00417-024-06628-1

[108] Menapace R, Findl O, Kriechbaum K, Leydolt-Koeppl C. Accommodating intraocular lenses: A critical review of present and future concepts. Graefe's Archive for Clinical and Experimental Ophthalmology. Apr 2007;**245**(4):473-489. DOI: 10.1007/s00417-006-0391-6

[109] Liang Y-L, Jia S-B. Clinical application of accommodating intraocular lens. International Journal of Ophthalmology. 2018;**11**(6):1028-1037. DOI: 10.18240/ijo.2018.06.22

[110] Kohl JC et al. Long-term uveal and capsular biocompatibility of a new accommodating intraocular lens. Journal of Cataract and Refractive Surgery. 2014;**40**(12):2113-2119. DOI: 10.1016/j.jcrs.2014.10.011

[111] Garg S, De Jesus MT, Fletcher LM, Chayet A, Barragán E, Casey P. Twelve-month clinical outcomes after implantation of a new, modular, anterior shape-changing fluid optic intraocular lens. Journal of Cataract & Refractive Surgery. Oct 2022;**48**(10):1134-1140. DOI: 10.1097/j.jcrs.0000000000000935

[112] Alvarez LW. Two-Element Variable-Power Spherical Lens. US3305294A. 1967. [Online]. Available from: https://patents.google.com/patent/US3305294A/en [Accessed: August 15, 2025]

[113] Alio JL et al. Visual outcomes and accommodative response of the Lumina accommodative intraocular lens. American Journal of Ophthalmology. Apr 2016;**164**:37-48. DOI: 10.1016/j.ajo.2016.01.006

[114] Alió JL et al. Analysis of accommodative performance of a new accommodative intraocular lens. Journal of Refractive Surgery. 2018;**34**(2):78-83. DOI: 10.3928/1081597X-20171205-01

[115] RayOne Galaxy Spiral IOL Launch Announced by Rayner. Ophthalmology Times. [Online]. Available from: https://www.ophthalmologytimes.com/view/rayone-galaxy-spiral-iol-launch-announced-by-rayner; [Accessed: August 04, 2025]

[116] Galinier L, Renaud-Goud P, Brusau J, Kergadallan L, Augereau J, Simon B. Spiral diopter: Freeform lenses with enhanced multifocal behavior. Optica. 2024;**11**(2):238-244. DOI: 10.1364/OPTICA.507066

[117] Tran. Rayner's Spiral Full-Range-of-Vision RayOne Galaxy IOL Debuts in India. CAKE. [Online]. Available from: https://cakemagazine.org/rayners-spiral-full-range-of-vision-rayone-galaxy-iol-debuts-in-india/; [Accessed: August 04, 2025]

[118] Moshirfar M et al. Astigmatic correction with implantation of a light adjustable vs monofocal lens: A single site analysis of a randomized controlled trial. International Journal of Ophthalmology. 2019;**12**(7):1101-1107. DOI: 10.18240/ijo.2019.07.08

[119] Jones M, Terveen DC, Berdahl JP, Thompson V, Kramer BA, Ferguson TJ.

Clinical outcomes of the light-adjustable lens in eyes with a history of prior corneal refractive surgery. Journal of Cataract and Refractive Surgery. 2024;**50**(9):936-941. DOI: 10.1097/j.jcrs.0000000000001481

[120] Brierley L. Refractive results after implantation of a light-adjustable intraocular lens in postrefractive surgery cataract patients. Ophthalmology. 2013;**120**(10):1968-1972. DOI: 10.1016/j.ophtha.2013.03.010

[121] Ang RET, Yoo P, Liu J. Visual outcomes after optic exchange of a modular intraocular lens. Journal of Cataract and Refractive Surgery. 2021;**47**(11):1441-1447. DOI: 10.1097/j.jcrs.0000000000000654

[122] Bozukova D et al. Improved performances of intraocular lenses by poly(ethylene glycol) chemical coatings. Biomacromolecules. 2007;**8**(8):2379-2387. DOI: 10.1021/bm0701649

[123] Wu KY, Khammar R, Sheikh H, Marchand M. Innovative polymeric biomaterials for intraocular lenses in cataract surgery. Journal of Functional Biomaterials. 2024;**15**(12):391. DOI: 10.3390/jfb15120391

[124] Nagy Z, Takacs A, Filkorn T, Sarayba M. Initial clinical evaluation of an intraocular femtosecond laser in cataract surgery. Journal of Refractive Surgery. 2009;**25**(12):1053-1060. DOI: 10.3928/1081597X-20091117-04

[125] Wu BM, Williams GP, Tan A, Mehta JS. A comparison of different operating systems for femtosecond lasers in cataract surgery. Journal of Ophthalmology. 2015;**2015**:616478. DOI: 10.1155/2015/616478

[126] Sun H, Fritz A, Dröge G, Neuhann T, Bille JF. Femtosecond-laser-assisted cataract surgery (FLACS). In: Bille JF, editor. High Resolution Imaging in Microscopy and Ophthalmology: New Frontiers in Biomedical Optics. Cham (CH): Springer; 2019. [Online]. Available from: http://www.ncbi.nlm.nih.gov/books/NBK554036/ [Accessed: August 04, 2025]

[127] Aristeidou A et al. The evolution of corneal and refractive surgery with the femtosecond laser. Eye and Vision. 2015;**2**(1):12. DOI: 10.1186/s40662-015-0022-6

[128] Chaves MAPD et al. Architecture evaluation of the main clear corneal incisions in femtosecond laser-assisted cataract surgery by optical coherence tomography imaging. Clinical Ophthalmology. 2019;**13**:365-372. DOI: 10.2147/OPTH.S184024

[129] Diakonis V et al. Comparison of surgically induced astigmatism between femtosecond laser and manual clear corneal incisions for cataract surgery. Journal of Cataract and Refractive Surgery. 2015;**41**:2075-2080. DOI: 10.1016/j.jcrs.2015.11.004

[130] Verdina T et al. Long-term evaluation of capsulotomy shape and posterior capsule opacification after low-energy bimanual femtosecond laser-assisted cataract surgery. Journal of Ophthalmology. 2020;**2020**:6431314. DOI: 10.1155/2020/6431314

[131] Reddy JC, Devta S, Vupparaboina KK, Ali MH, Vaddavalli PK. Early results of circularity and centration of capsulotomy prepared by three different methods. International Journal of Ophthalmology. Jan 2021;**14**(1):76-82. DOI: 10.18240/ijo.2021.01.11

[132] Whang W-J et al. Effect of pre-fragmentation on efficacy and safety

for phacoemulsification in femtosecond laser-assisted cataract surgery: A non-randomized clinical trial. Annals of Translational Medicine. 2023;**11**(1):5. DOI: 10.21037/atm-22-1279

[133] Pichardo-Loera NS, Corredor-Ortega C, Castro-Monreal MA, Massaro-Corredor MG, Pérez-Vázquez JF, Gonzalez-Salinas R. Femtosecond laser-assisted cataract surgery versus conventional phacoemulsification: A meta-analysis of randomized controlled trials. European Journal of Ophthalmology. 2024;**34**(5):1458-1468. DOI: 10.1177/11206721241229129

[134] Espaillat A, Pérez O, Potvin R. Clinical outcomes using standard phacoemulsification and femtosecond laser-assisted surgery with toric intraocular lenses. Clinical Ophthalmology. 2016;**10**:555-563. DOI: 10.2147/OPTH.S102083

[135] Kanclerz P, Alio JL. The benefits and drawbacks of femtosecond laser-assisted cataract surgery. European Journal of Ophthalmology. 2021;**31**(3):1021-1030. DOI: 10.1177/1120672120922448

[136] Refractive Error after Cataract Surgery. EyeWiki. [Online]. Available from: https://eyewiki.org/Refractive_Error_After_Cataract_Surgery#Etiology; [Accessed: August 04, 2025]

[137] Moshirfar M, McCaughey MV, Santiago-Caban L. Corrective techniques and future directions for treatment of residual refractive error following cataract surgery. Expert Review of Ophthalmology. 2014;**9**(6):529-537. DOI: 10.1586/17469899.2014.966817

[138] Fernández-Buenaga R, Alió JL, Pérez Ardoy AL, Quesada AL, Pinilla-Cortés L, Barraquer RI. Resolving refractive error after cataract surgery: IOL exchange, piggyback lens, or LASIK. Journal of Refractive Surgery. 2013;**29**(10):676-683. DOI: 10.3928/1081597X-20130826-01

[139] Kim P, Briganti EM, Sutton GL, Lawless MA, Rogers CM, Hodge C. Laser in situ keratomileusis for refractive error after cataract surgery. Journal of Cataract and Refractive Surgery. 2005;**31**(5):979-986. DOI: 10.1016/j.jcrs.2004.08.054

[140] Jin GJC, Merkley KH, Crandall AS, Jones YJ. Laser in situ keratomileusis versus lens-based surgery for correcting residual refractive error after cataract surgery. Journal of Cataract and Refractive Surgery. 2008;**34**(4):562-569. DOI: 10.1016/j.jcrs.2007.11.040

[141] Somani SN, Moshirfar M, Patel BC. Photorefractive keratectomy. In: StatPearls. Treasure Island (FL): StatPearls Publishing; 2025. [Online]. Available from: http://www.ncbi.nlm.nih.gov/books/NBK549887/ [Accessed: August 04, 2025]

[142] Rohlf D, La Nasa A, Terveen D, Shafer B, Thompson V, Berdahl J. Outcomes of LASIK vs PRK enhancement in eyes with prior cataract surgery. Journal of Cataract and Refractive Surgery. 2023;**49**(1):62-68. DOI: 10.1097/j.jcrs.0000000000001028

[143] Chang Y-M, Liang C-M, Weng T-H, Chien K-H, Lee C-H. Mitomycin C for the prevention of corneal haze in photorefractive keratectomy: A meta-analysis and trial sequential analysis. Acta Ophthalmologica. 2021;**99**(6):652-662. DOI: 10.1111/aos.14704

[144] Sekundo W, Kunert KS, Blum M. Small incision corneal refractive surgery using the small incision lenticule extraction (SMILE) procedure for the correction of myopia and myopic astigmatism: Results of a 6 month prospective study. The

British Journal of Ophthalmology. 2011;**95**(3):335-339. DOI: 10.1136/bjo.2009.174284

[145] Saad A, Klabe K, Kirca M, Kretz FAT, Auffarth G, Breyer DRH. Refractive outcomes of small lenticule extraction (SMILE) pro® with a 2 MHz femtosecond laser. International Ophthalmology. 2024;**44**(1):52. DOI: 10.1007/s10792-024-02915-2

[146] Semiz F, Lokaj AS, Musa NH, Semiz CE, Demirsoy ZA, Semiz O. SMILE for the treatment of residual refractive error after cataract surgery. Ophthalmology and Therapy. 2022;**11**(4):1539-1550. DOI: 10.1007/s40123-022-00526-7

[147] Abdelghany AA, Alio JL. Surgical options for correction of refractive error following cataract surgery. Eye and vision (London, England). 2014;**1**:2. DOI: 10.1186/s40662-014-0002-2

[148] Gundersen KG, Potvin R. A review of results after implantation of a secondary intraocular lens to correct residual refractive error after cataract surgery. Clinical Ophthalmology. 2017;**11**:1791-1796. DOI: 10.2147/OPTH.S144675

[149] Khoramnia R, Kahraman G, Amon M, Łabuz G, Baur ID, Auffarth GU. Polypseudophakia: From 'piggyback' to supplementary sulcus-fixated IOLs. Graefe's Archive for Clinical and Experimental Ophthalmology. 2025;**263**(3):603-624. DOI: 10.1007/s00417-024-06618-3

[150] Zhang L et al. Comparison of visual Neuroadaptations after multifocal and Monofocal intraocular lens implantation. Frontiers in Neuroscience. 2021;**15**:648863. DOI: 10.3389/fnins.2021.648863

[151] Schor C, Landsman L, Erickson P. Ocular dominance and the interocular suppression of blur in monovision. American Journal of Optometry and Physiological Optics. 1987;**64**(10):723-730. DOI: 10.1097/00006324-198710000-00002

[152] Alió JL, Pikkel J. Multifocal Intraocular Lenses: Neuroadaptation. In: Alió JL, Pikkel J, editors. Multifocal Intraocular Lenses: The Art and the Practice. Cham: Springer International Publishing; 2019. pp. 53-60. DOI: 10.1007/978-3-030-21282-7_5

[153] Nishi Y, Nishi H, Fukui M, Tatsumichi M, Nishi K, Nishi O. Clinical assessment of brain adaptation following multifocal intraocular lens implantation. BMC Ophthalmology. 2025;**25**:116. DOI: 10.1186/s12886-025-03955-7

[154] Kaymak H, Fahle M, Ott G, Mester U. Intraindividual comparison of the effect of training on visual performance with ReSTOR and Tecnis diffractive multifocal IOLs. Journal of Refractive Surgery. 2008;**24**(3):287-293. DOI: 10.3928/1081597X-20080301-11

[155] Al-Shymali O, Alió Del Barrio JL, McAlinden C, Canto M, Primavera L, Alio JL. Multifocal intraocular lens exchange to monofocal for the management of neuroadaptation failure. Eye and vision (London, England). 2022;**9**(1):40. DOI: 10.1186/s40662-022-00311-4

[156] Alió F, Barraquer R, Cantó-Cerdán M, Alió JL. Causes of intraocular pseudophakic lens explantation in Spain. European Journal of Ophthalmology. 2024;**34**(2):432-439. DOI: 10.1177/11206721231187921

Chapter 5

Optical Coherence Tomography in Cataract Surgery

Adel Ebraheem

Abstract

Utilizing optical coherence tomography (OCT) before and after cataract surgery is critical for optimal outcomes. Complications following cataract surgery are frequently observed, including conditions such as Irvine Gass syndrome, uveitis, elevated intraocular pressure and several others. Additionally, ophthalmologists may carry out cataract surgery on patients who have other eye conditions, including wet age-related macular degeneration, macular holes, epiretinal membrane, glaucoma and several other ocular diseases. Utilizing anterior and posterior segment OCT enables the surgeon to manage complications efficiently and provide the patient with an accurate prognosis and follow up management plan. Additionally, intraoperative OCT can be employed during cataract surgery to address specific situations, including those arising from ocular trauma complicated by intraocular foreign bodies and membrane peeling.

Keywords: ocular coherence tomography, cataract, anterior segment, intraocular lens, intraocular lens power formulas

1. Introduction

Optical Coherence Tomography (OCT) is a non-invasive diagnostic technique that produces cross-sectional images of the retina. It uses the principle of interferometry to create detailed images of the retinal structure, achieving a precision of at least 10–15 microns.

In the early stages, OCT image acquisition was performed using a time-domain technology achieving a speed of approximately 400 A-scans per second, distributed across six radial slices, each separated by 30 degrees. Spectral-domain technology, in contrast, performs scans at a rate of approximately 20,000–40,000 A-scans per second.

A higher frequency and greater volume of scans reduce the likelihood of motion artifacts, enhance image resolution, and increase the probability of identifying lesions. The application of spectral domain technology, through enhanced depth imaging (EDI), enables a more detailed visualization of the choroid and the underlying layers.

The implementation of swept-source technology has primarily driven the latest developments in optical coherence tomography. This technology utilizes a wavelength-sweeping laser, along with a dual-balanced photodetector. This technology results in a remarkable enhancement in acquisition speeds, allowing for the collection of 100,000–400,000 A-scans per second. The improved axial resolution and accelerated scanning rates contribute to superior image averaging, thus enhancing image quality and enabling a more thorough investigation of deeper structures.

Swept-source optical coherence tomography (SS-OCT) has been employed to produce non-invasive, dye-free OCT angiography. In conclusion, OCT angiography leverages motion contrast by assessing the decorrelation signal between several B-scans obtained at each retinal cross-section to identify blood flow.

To ensure a successful cataract surgery outcome, the OCT is currently used in preoperative assessment, intraoperative guidance, and postoperative follow-up to detect any potential complications. The OCT allows detailed visualization of the anterior chamber structure and retinal layers.

The objective of contemporary cataract surgery includes the correction of refractive errors and the optimization of optical quality by decreasing high-order aberrations. Recently, a proposal has been made to tailor the design of intraocular lenses to the unique anatomical parameters of each patient [1]. Yet, the accuracy of intraocular lens (IOL) power selection is limited by the precision of pre-operative ocular biometry and the approximations that are applied in the IOL calculation formulas [2].

In general, theoretical calculations for IOL power, including the SRK-T method, adopt a thin lens framework and apply different approximations for the cornea and lens, usually within the paraxial domain.

To utilize these formulas, it is essential to have preoperative data related to axial length and corneal power, along with an estimation of the postoperative anterior chamber depth (ACD), commonly referred to as Estimated Lens Position (ELP).

The precise ray tracing method can be utilized, which requires positional and geometrical data related to the cornea and crystalline lens [3].

Higher-order aberrations in pseudophakic eyes can be predicted using individualized computer simulations that factor in the position of intraocular pressure (IOP), corneal topography, and the depth of the anterior chamber [4].

Furthermore, acquiring three-dimensional data on the crystalline lens and the anatomy of the anterior chamber is crucial for improving the accuracy of the estimated postoperative effective lens position. Currently, there is no device available that offers an exhaustive and complete optical analysis of the anterior segment, which is imperative for the effective planning of cataract surgery.

Spectral OCT equips surgeons with unparalleled lateral and axial resolution three-dimensional imaging of the anterior segment. This advanced technology enhances precision and confidence in surgical procedures, ultimately fostering better patient outcomes.

2. Corneal architecture and pathology

The curvature of the cornea contributes to about 72 percent of the total eye power. A significant limitation of using keratometry in the evaluation of cataract surgery is that it fails to offer enough data on corneal topography outside the central 3 mm. Computerized videokeratography is the most reliable device that provides standardized corneal topography results [5].

A review of over 260,000 eyes found that fewer than 1% of cataract surgeons achieved an accuracy of ±0.50 D at or above 92%. Moreover, most surgeons had an accuracy level around 78% [6]. It is indisputable that disorders of the cornea and diseases impacting the ocular surface considerably influence visual acuity results.

The likelihood of corneal healing complications and decompensation after cataract surgery increases when corneal thickness is above 640 microns and in the presence of corneal dystrophy.

Izatt et al. first described anterior segment optical coherence tomography (ASOCT) imaging in 1994, utilizing the same wavelength of light as that used in retinal OCT, which is 830 nm [7]. This wavelength does not provide an optimal visualization of the anterior chamber angle because of its restricted penetration through the scleral tissue. Subsequently, a longer wavelength of 1310 nm presents improved penetration and the ability for real-time imaging at a rate of 8 frames per second [8].

The most superficial, thin, hyperreflective layer identified by AS-OCT is the tear film. A number of researchers utilized AS-OCT to examine the corneal endothelium and tear film in patients diagnosed with systemic lupus erythematosus; their findings indicated that these patients exhibited a reduced tear meniscus and a decrease in central corneal thickness. Moreover, the scientist discovered that patients with systemic lupus had a decreased tear meniscus thickness even without exhibiting dry eye clinical features [9].

With AS-OCT, practitioners can accurately map clear and opacified corneas, facilitating the precise delineation of the various corneal layers. A variety of corneal disorders, such as infectious, inflammatory, or ectatic conditions, can be evaluated with greater precision through the use of AS-OCT. The measurement tool aids in the assessment of the advancement or resolution of subepithelial infiltrates, corneal scars, or edema (**Figure 1**) [10].

Pachymetry, corneal topography, and Scheimpflug imaging are employed in the diagnosis of ectatic conditions. The advent of AS-OCT allows specialists to observe and monitor the distinct characteristics of keratoconus across the different layers of the cornea. Recent research has underscored the pivotal role of Bowman's membrane and epithelial thickness maps at the apex of the cone in effectively differentiating non-diseased eyes from those affected by manifest, subclinical, and forme fruste keratoconus.

The cataract surgeon should create a clear cornea incision (CCI) architecture to ensure successful phacoemulsification. The ophthalmologist strives to prevent various complications, such as wound leakage and Descemet's membrane detachment, resulting from misconstruction of CCIs. The AS-OCT can be used for further evaluation of CCI parameters such as incision angle, location, and length, along with associated factors, including posterior wound gap and wound retraction during the initial postoperative period [11].

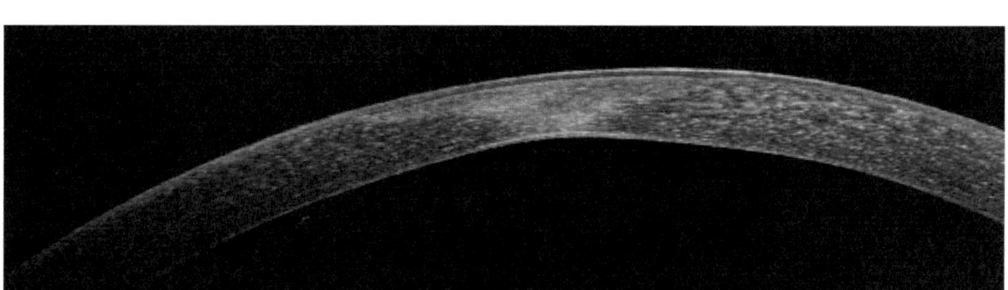

Figure 1.
Anterior segment ocular coherence tomography shows corneal scar.

Several research surgeons found that AS-OCT revealed various types of Descemet's membrane detachment, including planar and nonplanar, as well as local and extensive [12].

The literature features anecdotal reports on the use of OCT-assisted Descemetopexy during surgery for non-resolving Descemet's membrane detachments [12]. Furthermore, this device is beneficial for selecting the right treatment options and for evaluating treatment outcomes when corneal edema is identified. The OCT serves to guide cataract surgeons in choosing the right instruments for corneal incisions and the relevant surgical techniques, especially when they should endeavor to avoid making corneal incisions in vascularized regions, if possible. The cataract surgeon is required to document the placement of radial or astigmatic incisions, as well as any evident issues with the healing process [13].

The ray tracing equation utilizes a specific technique, like the Oslen formula, which follows the path of refracted light from the surfaces of the cornea and lens. By implementing this approach, one can account for high-order aberrations to achieve enhanced accuracy [14].

The AS-OCT is used in evaluating the anatomical stability of the implanted keratoprosthesis, as it visualizes the interface between the cornea and the anterior keratoprosthesis [15].

3. Anterior angle, crystalline lens, and its anterior capsule and zonules

Through the evaluation of AS-OCT images, the scleral spur is recognized as an inwardly directed projection of the sclera at the point where the inner curvature of the sclera intersects with the curvature of the cornea. The apposition of the iris to the inner corneo-scleral wall is utilized as a qualitative means for detecting angle closure; however, it is imperative to note that the level of apposition can vary and does not directly correlate with angle closure as defined by gonioscopy [16].

The AS-OCT software built in is capable of quantitatively assessing the anterior chamber angle, which requires identification of the scleral spur. A variety of quantitative assessment metrics are available for the anterior angle

1. Angle opening distance (in mm): Defined as the perpendicular distance between a point that is 500 μm (AOD 500) or 750 μm (AOD 750) anterior to the scleral spur and the iris on the opposite side.

2. Angle recess area (in mm^2): The triangular section (ARA 500 or 750) enclosed by the AOD 500 or 750, the front surface of the iris, and the inner corneo-scleral wall

3. The area of the trabecular space (measured in mm^2) is defined as the trapezoidal area (TISA 500 or 750) enclosed by the AOD 500 or 750, the anterior surface of the iris, the inner wall of the corneoscleral region, and the perpendicular distance from the scleral spur to the opposing iris (**Figure 2**)

Due to corneal abnormalities or a lack of cooperation from the patient, ASOCT serves as a substitute of gonioscopy in clinical glaucoma practice. OCT's non-contact nature enhances patient comfort while providing accurate assessments of the angle. The OCT offers better visualization of the anterior angle than gonioscopy, especially in low illumination due to physiological mydriasis. The Ultrasound microscopy

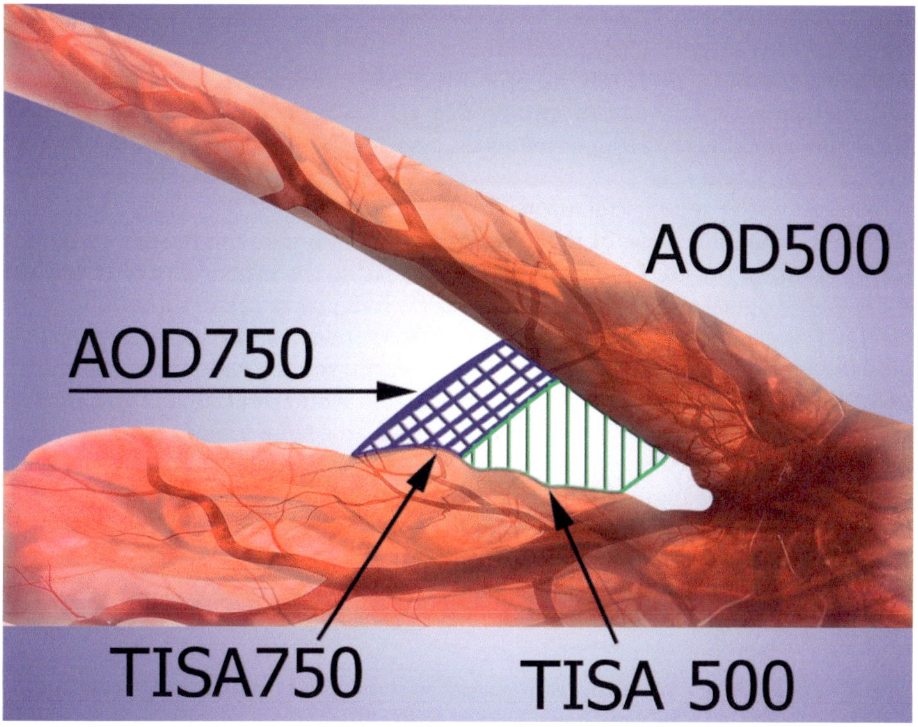

Figure 2.
Anterior chamber angle anatomical landmarks and measurement of AOD, and TISA in an optical coherence tomography line scan image.

is superior to AS_OCT in the diagnosis of conditions such as iridociliary lesion or plateau iris that are associated with angle closure.

Primary angle closure suspect (PACS) is characterized by a narrow angle that is at risk of angle closure. Trabecular obstruction as a result of angle closure is the hallmark of primary angle closure (PAC). If optic neuropathy is the result of PAC, the condition is called primary angle closure glaucoma (PACO). The majority of ophthalmologists choose phacoemulsification and IOL implantation as the primary intervention for PACG.

Cataract surgeons recommend using capsular rings or scleral-fixed IOL in case of lens zonule instability or weakness, which are often associated with primary angle closure [17].

The preliminary signs of lens subluxation due to partial zonular dehiscence include iridodonesis, phacodonesis, the visibility of the lens equator, and an asymmetric ACD. It is challenging to determine zonular instability through slit-lamp, gonioscopy, or ocular B-mode ultrasound in the case of PAC, as malposition of the crystalline lens is not always apparent in eyes with shallow ACD.

The AS-OCT showed the ability to identify zonular instability post-acute angle closure attack. The eyes with zonular instability are characterized by diminished hyperopic spherical equivalent, longer axial length, shallower anterior chamber depth, and increased lens vault [18].

Pei and others observed that the crystalline lens is characterized by steeper anterior curvature, increased thickness in the anterior portion, and elevated ratio of anterior-to-posterior portion thickness in patient with PAC diseases [19].

Sometimes the AS-OCT is used intraoperatively during cataract surgery accompanied by glaucoma surgery [20].

There are presently three microscope-integrated commercial intraoperative OCT (iOCT) platforms that have been approved by the US Food and Drug Administration (FDA)—these include the Haag-Streit iOCT system, the Zeiss Rescan 700, and the Leica EnFocus system [21].

In patients with pseudoexfoliation, the high-resolution OCT enables the identification of increased thickness of the anterior capsule compared to normal individuals [22]. Additionally, the OCT is significant in evaluating the probability of IOL tilting after cataract surgery and in the analysis of toric IOL power calculations [23].

AS-OCT-assisted Descemet striping automated endothelial keratoplasty was applied in managing the anterior chamber fibrous ingrowth. A surgical operation assisted by AS OCT was conducted on a 61-year-old woman suffering from corneal edema and chronic angle-closure glaucoma, which arose due to fibrous ingrowth after two glaucoma shunt device implantations. The procedure involved the dissection and removal of the fibrous ingrowth in the anterior chamber, in addition to DSAEK. The recovery period post-surgery was uncomplicated, resulting in a positive outcome [24].

4. Posterior capsule

The lens capsule is a smooth, transparent basement membrane that varies in thickness between 2 and 28 microns, surrounding the entire crystalline lens. The lens capsule is made of type IV collagen and glycosaminoglycans.

One of the possible complications during cataract surgery is posterior capsule rupture, which requires careful evaluation of the capsule. Some surgeons use AS-OCT in evaluating the integrity of the posterior capsular bag. It was found that the sensitivity and specificity of AS-OCT in identifying posterior capsule dehiscence were 100% and 94.92%, respectively [25]. A different study revealed that AS-OCT achieved approximately 94% accuracy in assessing the morphological features of cataracts. Additionally, the OCT identified fibrosis and ruptures in both the anterior and posterior capsules with an accuracy exceeding 95% [26].

A group of researchers at the Vienna Institute for Research in Ocular Surgery observed that employing the AS-OCT intraoperatively for lens capsule measurement improves the predictability of IOL position post-surgery rather than relying on preoperative ACD measurements [27].

One of the rare complications of post-cataract surgery is capsular block syndrome (CBS), which is characterized by a collection between the capsular bag and the IOL. Fluid retention between the IOP and posterior capsule is the result of impairment of aqueous humor exchange between the anterior chamber and the capsular bag. Researchers observed that persistent capsulorhexis and adhesion of the anterior capsule to the IOL are the leading causes of capsular block syndrome. A range of manifestations associated with CBS has been documented, such as reduced visual clarity, increased ocular pressure, closed-angle glaucoma, and posterior capsule rupture.

The evolution of ophthalmic imaging technology allows for a definitive diagnosis through Scheimpflug-based photography, AS-OCT, or anterior segment UBM. While Scheimpflug-based photography offers valuable anterior chamber insights, spectral domain AS-OCT delivers superior detail about the intraocular lens (IOL) and any fluid between the IOL and the posterior capsular bag, leading to improved assessments and patient outcomes [28].

DOI: http://dx.doi.org/10.5772/intechopen.1013172

5. Vitreous and retina

The presence of occult macular pathologies that remain undetected through biomicroscopic fundus examination is significant in assessing the final visual acuity of patients post-cataract surgery. The OCT serves as a crucial imaging technique for diagnosing and monitoring both clinical and subclinical macular lesions. This highlights the critical role OCT plays in preoperative evaluations, as 13.7% of patients were found to have undetected macular issues that could influence their postoperative visual outcomes [29].

Velthoven et al. observed that the presence of cataract compromised the quality of the OCT image, and macular thickness was increased after cataract surgery [30].

Recognizing retinal pathology promptly yields three crucial benefits: (1) It equips the patient with a solid prognosis prior to surgery. (2) Specific retinal disorders, including macular oedema, must be managed before cataract surgery. (3) The presence of serious macular or optic nerve diseases can result in the cancelation of cataract surgery.

Studies that tracked the frequency of macular pathology also provided descriptions of the types of pathology that were observed. These pathologies were broadly categorized into five groups: interface abnormalities, macular degeneration, oedema, macular hole, and miscellaneous.

One of the most common retinal interface irregularities is associated with the epiretinal membrane (ERM). It is a notable challenge to diagnose fine ERM without OCT screening [31]. The existence of ERM entails a heightened risk for the development of cystoid macular edema subsequent to intraocular surgery [32]. Cystoid macular edema is regarded as one of the most prevalent complications that hinder recovery, extend the duration of treatment, and necessitate more intensive therapeutic interventions [33].

Following the enrollment of 614 patients for pre-cataract surgery assessment, the OCT identified retinal pathology in approximately 7% of individuals who exhibited a normal fundoscopic examination. Among these, 5% were diagnosed with ERM, age-related macular degeneration was observed in 7 eyes, an intraretinal cyst was found in less than 1%, a lamellar hole was present in 4 patients, and a full-thickness hole was noted in one eye [34].

In a large-scale cohort study from China, OCT detected macular pathologies in 25% of the assessed eyes. While AMD, central serous chorioretinopathy, and polypoidal choroidal vasculopathy were the least frequently reported conditions, the three most common macular pathologies found were ERM, myopic atrophy, and dome-shaped macula associated with pathological myopia [31].

Kowallick et al. documented the presence of drusen bodies in four out of 162 eyes, as well as retinal pigment epithelial atrophy in one eye, during their examination of the patients' OCT scans. They hypothesized that the low prevalence could be attributed to the significant cataract densities observed in the patients involved in their study (**Figure 3**) [35].

In patients with macular pathologies, multifocal or trifocal intraocular lenses may fail to deliver optimal visual outcomes, potentially leading to a decrease in contrast sensitivity [36].

Swept source OCT is superior to SD-OCT by utilizing longer wavelengths and a faster scanning speed [37]. Theoretically, The SS-OCT provides higher-resolution images compared to SD-OCT, which might reveal subtle macular pathologies [38]. In contrast, the fovea scan produced by SS-OCT exhibits a flatter profile when

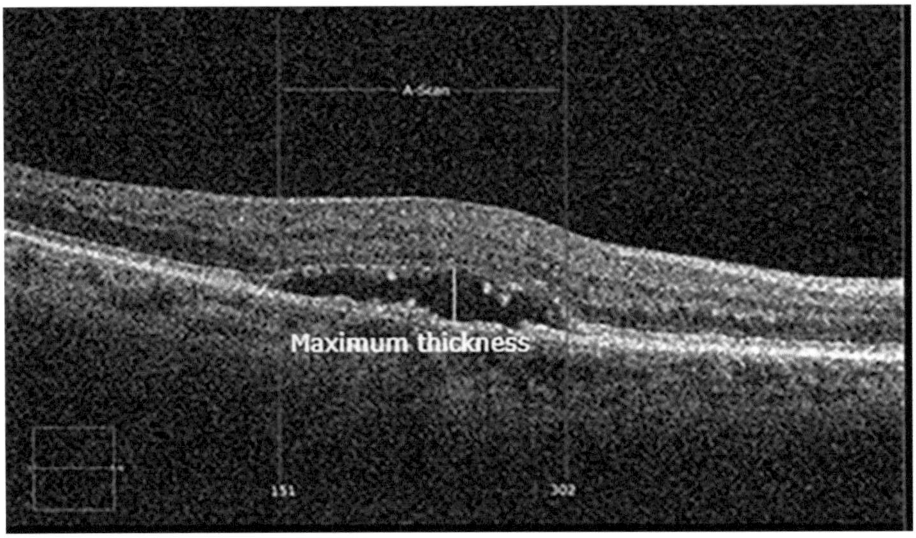

Figure 3.
Ocular coherence tomography shows subretinal fluid with intraretinal hyperintensity foci.

compared to that of SD-OCT, resulting in a reduced scan area of 1 mm. Consequently, the sensitivity of macular screening may not be equivalent to that of SD-OCT [38]. In their study, Hirnschall et al. found that the SS-OCT biometer had a moderate sensitivity of 0.48 to 0.62 when compared to SD-OCT, identifying macular pathology in about 58.5% of eyes that SD-OCT revealed macular pathology [39] The subsequent research carried out by Tognetto et al. clearly demonstrated that the SS-OCT biometer attained a mean sensitivity of 0.81 when compared to SD-OCT. It successfully identified pathology in 81% of eyes that were deemed abnormal based on SD-OCT findings [40].

It was demonstrated that the SS-OCT is just as effective as the SD-OCT in identifying macular holes and intraretinal fluid by a study conducted by Hirnschall et al. However, the SS-OCT scan was not effective in detecting geographic atrophy and epiretinal membranes (ERM). The authors proposed that widening the SS-OCT scan to a diameter of 1 mm may result in an improvement in image sensitivity [39].

6. Intraocular lens power calculation

An accurate assessment of ocular dimensions is crucial for surgical intervention, especially cataract and refractive surgeries. Axial length measurement is critical for the calculation of IOL power following cataract surgery. The assessment of axial length through non-contact biometry devices outperforms the traditional ultrasound method by effectively resolving issues related to variability and ocular indentation.

To significantly reduce refractive prediction errors, it is imperative to accurately predict postoperative optical biometry using preoperative data. Research by Norrby and colleagues illustrates that predicting the position of the IOL prior to surgery can result in notable inaccuracies in determining the appropriate IOL power [41]. The calculation of IOL power relies heavily on the postoperative ACD, known as ELP, which varies depending on the specific formula applied. Unfortunately, this approach often fails to capture the true postoperative ACD from an anatomical perspective.

This limitation is especially pronounced in third-generation IOL power calculation, specifically, Hoffer Q7 [42], Holladay 1 [43], and SRK/T [44].

Ray tracing software can determine the IOL power with more accuracy through a precise estimation pf postoperative ACD. The methodology proposed by Goto et al. focuses on predicting postoperative ACD, utilizing the angle-to-angle (ATA) depth derived from AS–OCT [45]. Enriquez et al. introduced a technique that facilitates precise estimation and quantification of the complete shape of the crystalline lens obtained from OCT data. They emphasized that the preoperative anterior segment parameters are vital for accurately estimating the IOL position [46].

A research conducted by Satou et al. aimed at creating a novel formula utilizing paraxial ray tracing for IOL power calculations, incorporating postoperative IOL placements, and assessing the precision of this newly formulated equation.

The enrolled patients were organized into training and validating subgroups. The alignment of the implanted IOLs in the training dataset was rigorously evaluated through multiple linear regression analyses, conducted one month after the surgical procedures. The validation dataset successfully computed postoperative refractive values using paraxial ray tracing of both the cornea and lens. This methodology was based on assumptions regarding finite structural thicknesses and unique surface curvatures. The new formula demonstrated a percentage error of around 84%, which falls within ±0.50 diopters. The formula improved predictions of postoperative refraction and may be useful for eyes with abnormal characteristics, such as unusual corneal curvatures and varying axial lengths [47].

A group of researchers investigated the application of OCT for evaluating corneal power and improving the selection of IOL power during cataract surgeries after refractive surgery. A comprehensive analysis of 46 patients demonstrated that all underwent uncomplicated cataract surgery with the successful implantation of monofocal IOLs. The mean arithmetic prediction error for postoperative refraction was recorded as 0.05 ± 0.65 D for the OCT formula, 0.14 ± 0.83 D for the Haigis-L formula, and 0.24 ± 0.82 D for the Shammas-PL formula in cases with no prior history. In eyes that have had laser vision correction, OCT-based IOL power calculation demonstrated greater predictive accuracy compared to the Haigis-L and Shammas-PL formulas [48].

Savini et al. focused on evaluating the results of IOL power calculations, employing data gathered through a SS-OCT optical biometer. They concluded that the SS-OCT optical biometer's measurements contribute to the precise calculation of IOL power, as all formulas yielded a prediction error within 0.50 D in at least 80% of patients [49].

7. Cost-effectiveness and the future of OCT in cataract surgery

Several surgeons advocate for the OCT screening in patients being assessed for cataract surgery, especially those considering premium IOLs. This approach aims to refine patient selection criteria and ultimately improve postoperative satisfaction outcomes. The OCT screening reimbursement is not guaranteed unless the patient has a reasonable medical diagnosis according to Medicare and Medicaid Services guidelines.

In individuals exhibiting normal OCT results, the direct medical expenses and lost opportunity costs may be incurred by the physician or the medical institution. Given the current uncertainty regarding the cost-effectiveness of a preoperative OCT in cataract surgery, it is likely that patients who pay out-of-pocket for multifocal IOLs represent the subgroup most affected by and most dissatisfied with undiagnosed retinal pathologies.

For individuals evaluating cataract surgery, the performance of optical coherence tomography with an IOL before the operation may raise the overall costs. However, it may also help uncover other macular conditions and improve life quality. The cost of an OCT that is reimbursable by Medicare was $41.81, with all associated costs and benefits adjusted for inflation to reflect 2019 U.S. dollars, discounted at a rate of 3% per year over 16 years. In the fundamental scenario, an adjunctive preoperative OCT proved to be cost-effective from both a third-party payer and societal viewpoint in the United States. The study indicated that 64.4% of patients would likely accept the extra cost of an OCT prior to cataract surgery, considering a willingness-to-pay standard of $50,000 for each quality-adjusted life year [50].

Many cataract surgeons will use OCT intraoperatively in patients who have an underlying anterior segment condition to achieve optimal visual outcomes.

Author details

Adel Ebraheem
Ophthalmology and Visual Sciences Department, University of Maryland—School of Medicine, USA

*Address all correspondence to: dr.adel.ebraheem@gmail.com

References

[1] Bellucci R, Morselli S. Optimizing higher-order aberrations with intraocular lens technology. Current Opinion in Ophthalmology. 2007;**18**(1):67-73. DOI: 10.1097/icu.0b013e3280121af1

[2] Norrby S. Sources of error in intraocular lens power calculation. Journal of Cataract and Refractive Surgery. 2008;**34**(3):368-376. DOI: 10.1016/j.jcrs.2007.10.03

[3] Preussner PR, Wahl J, Lahdo H, Dick B, Findl O. Ray tracing for intraocular lens calculation. Journal of Cataract and Refractive Surgery. 2002;**28**(8):1412-1419. DOI: 10.1016/s0886-3350(01)01346-3

[4] Rosales P, Marcos S. Customized computer models of eyes with intraocular lenses. Optics Express. 2007;**15**(5):2204-2218. DOI: 10.1364/OE.15.002204

[5] Howes FW. Patient workup for cataract surgery. In: Yanoff M, Duke J, editors. Ophthalmology. 4th ed. Elsevier Shop. Available from: https://shop.elsevier.com/books/ophthalmology/yanoff/978-1-4557-3984-4 [Accessed: November 05, 2025]

[6] Koch DD et al. Pursuing perfection in intraocular lens calculations: I. Logical Approach for classifying IOL calculation formulas. Journal of Cataract and Refractive Surgery. Jun 2017;**43**(6):717-718. DOI: 10.1016/j.jcrs.2017.06.006

[7] Izatt JA, Hee MR, Swanson EA, et al. Micrometer-scale resolution imaging of the anterior eye in vivo with optical coherence tomography. Archives of Ophthalmology. 1994;**112**:1584-1589

[8] Radhakrishnan S, Rollins AM, Roth JE, et al. Real-time optical coherence tomography of the anterior segment at 1310 nm. Archives of Ophthalmology. 2001;**119**:1179-1185

[9] Mahmoud MSE, Hamid MA, Abdelkader MF. Anterior segment optical coherence tomography of tear film and cornea in systemic lupus erythematosus patients. Clinical Ophthalmology. 2021;**15**:3391-3399. DOI: 10.2147/OPTH.S323673

[10] Konstantopoulos A, Kuo J, Anderson A, Hossain P. Assessment of the use of anterior segment optical coherence tomography in microbial keratitis. American Journal of Ophthalmology. 2008;**146**(4):534-542

[11] Wang L, Dixit L, Weikert MP, Jenkins RB, Koch DD. Healing changes in clear corneal cataract incisions evaluated using Fourier-domain optical coherence tomography. Journal of Cataract and Refractive Surgery. 2012;**38**:660-665

[12] Zhou SY, Wang CX, Cai XY, Liu YZ. Anterior segment OCT-based diagnosis and management of descemet's membrane detachment. Ophthalmologica. 2012;**227**:215-222. DOI: 10.1159/000334946

[13] Lee H, Kim EK, Kim HS, Kim TI. Fourier-domain optical coherence tomography evaluation of clear corneal incision structure according to blade material. Journal of Cataract and Refractive Surgery. 2014;**40**:1615-1624. DOI: 10.1016/j.jcrs.2014.01.036

[14] Olsen T, Hoffmann P. C constant: New concept for ray tracing-assisted intraocular lens power calculation. Journal of Cataract and Refractive Surgery. 2014;**40**(5):764-773. DOI: 10.1016/j.jcrs.2013.10.037

[15] Zarei-Ghanavati S, Betancurt C, Mas AM, Wang J, Perez VL. Ultra high resolution optical coherence tomography in Boston type I keratoprosthesis. Journal of Ophthalmic and Vision Research. 2015;**10**:26-32. DOI: 10.4103/2008-322X.156092

[16] Lavanya R, Foster PJ, Sakata LM, et al. Screening for narrow angle s in the Singapore population: Evaluation of new non-contact screening methods. Ophthalmology. 2008;**115**:1720-1727

[17] Kwon J, Sung KR. Factors associated with zonular instability during cataract surgery in eyes with acute angle closure attack. American Journal of Ophthalmology. 2017;**183**:118-124

[18] Pei X-T, Wang S-H, Qing G-P. Zonular instability-associated morphologic features in eyes with primary angle closure disease using the swept-source anterior segment—Optical coherence tomography system. BMC Ophthalmology. 2024;**24**:203. DOI: 10.1186/s12886-024-03462-1

[19] Pei XT, Wang SH, Qing GP, et al. Zonular instability-associated morphologic features in eyes with primary angle closure disease using the swept-source anterior segment—optical coherence tomography system. BMC Ophthalmology. 2024;**24**(1):203. Published 2024 Apr 30. DOI: 10.1186/s12886-024-03462-1

[20] Ang BCH, Lim SY, Dorairaj S. Intra-operative optical coherence tomography in glaucoma surgery—A systematic review. Eye (London, England). 2020;**34**(1):168-177. DOI: 10.1038/s41433-019-0689-3

[21] Posarelli C, Sartini F, Casini G, et al. What is the impact of intraoperative microscope-integrated OCT in ophthalmic surgery? Relevant applications and outcomes. A systematic review. Journal of Clinical Medicine. 2020;**9**(6):1682. DOI: 10.3390/jcm9061682

[22] Batur M, Seven E, Tekin S, Yasar T. Anterior lens capsule and iris thicknesses in pseudoexfoliation syndrome. Current Eye Research. 2017;**14**:1-5. DOI: 10.1080/02713683.2017.1338349

[23] Hirnschall N, Buehren T, Bajramovic F, Trost M, Teuber T, Findl O, et al. Prediction of postoperative intraocular lens tilt using swept-source optical coherence tomography. Journal of Cataract and Refractive Surgery. 2017;**43**:732-736. DOI: 10.1016/j.jcrs.2017.01.026

[24] Shazly TA, To LK, Conner IP, Espandar L. Intraoperative optical coherence tomography-assisted descemet stripping automated endothelial keratoplasty for anterior chamber fibrous ingrowth. Cornea. 2017;**36**(6):757-758. DOI: 10.1097/ICO.0000000000001192

[25] Pavan Kumar G, Krishnamurthy P, Nath M, Baskaran P, Janani M, Venkatesh R. Can preoperative anterior segment optical coherence tomography predict posterior capsule rupture during phacoemulsification in patients with posterior polar cataract? Journal of Cataract and Refractive Surgery. 2018;**44**(12):1441-1445. DOI: 10.1016/j.jcrs.2018.07.056. Epub 2018 Sep 18

[26] Bhardwaj A, Kaur S, Sukhija J, Gupta PC, Ram J. Role of swept-source anterior segment optical coherence tomography in imaging pediatric cataract. Indian Journal of Ophthalmology. 2023;**71**(5):2132-2138. DOI: 10.4103/IJO.IJO_2734_22

[27] Hirnschall N, Amir-Asgari S, Maedel S, Findl O. Predicting the postoperative intraocular lens position

using continuous intraoperative optical coherence tomography measurements. Investigative Ophthalmology & Visual Science. 2013;**54**(8):5196-5203. DOI: 10.1167/iovs.13-11991

[28] Wang X, Dong J, Zhang S, Sun B. OCT Application Before and After Cataract Surgery. London, UK: InTech; 2018. pp. 175-189. DOI: 10.5772/intechopen.77281

[29] Ahmed TM, Siddiqui MAR, Hussain B. Optical coherence tomography as a diagnostic intervention before cataract surgery-a review. Eye (London, England). 2023;**37**(11):2176-2182

[30] van Velthoven ME, van der Linden MH, de Smet MD, Faber DJ, Verbraak FD. Influence of cataract on optical coherence tomography image quality and retinal thickness. The British Journal of Ophthalmology. 2006;**90**(10):1259-1262. DOI: 10.1136/bjo.2004.097022. Erratum in: Br J Ophthalmol. 2010;94(12):1695

[31] Huang X, Zhang Z, Wang J, Meng X, Chen T, Wu Z. Macular assessment of preoperative optical coherence tomography in ageing Chinese undergoing routine cataract surgery. Scientific Reports. 2018;**8**:5103

[32] Hardin JS, Gauldin DW, Soliman MK, Chu CJ, Yang YC, Sallam AB. Cataract surgery outcomes in eyes with primary epiretinal membrane. JAMA Ophthalmology. 2018;**136**:148-154

[33] Han JV, Patel DV, Squirrell D, McGhee CN. Cystoid macular oedema following cataract surgery: A review. Clinical & Experimental Ophthalmology. 2019;**47**:346-356

[34] Pinto WP, Rabello LP, Ventura MC, Rocha CS, Ventura BV. Prevalence of macular abnormalities identified only by optical coherence tomography in Brazilian patients with cataract. Journal of Cataract and Refractive Surgery. 2019;**45**(7):915-918

[35] Kowallick A, Fischer CV, Hoerauf H. Optical coherence tomography findings in patients prior to cataract surgery regarded as unremarkable with ophthalmoscopy. PLoS One. 2018;**13**(12):e0208980

[36] Klein BR, Brown EN, Casden RS. Preoperative macular spectral-domain optical coherence tomography in patients considering advanced-technology intraocular lenses for cataract surgery. Journal of Cataract and Refractive Surgery. 2016;**42**:537-541

[37] Adhi M, Duker JS. Optical coherence tomography—Current and future applications. Current Opinion in Ophthalmology. 2013;**24**:213-221

[38] Goldhardt R, Rosen BS. Optical coherence tomography: Critical tool to manage expectations after cataract extraction. Current Ophthalmology Reports. 2020;**8**:129-135

[39] Hirnschall N, Leisser C, Radda S, Maedel S, Findl O. Macular disease detection with a swept-source optical coherence tomography-based biometry device in patients scheduled for cataract surgery. Journal of Cataract and Refractive Surgery. 2016;**42**:530-536

[40] Tognetto D, Pastore MR, De Giacinto C, Merli R, Franzon M, D'Aloisio R, et al. Swept- source optical coherence tomography biometer as screening strategy for macular disease in patients scheduled for cataract surgery. Scientific Reports. 2019;**9**:9912

[41] Norrby S. Sources of error in intraocular lens power calculation. Journal of Cataract and Refractive Surgery. 2008;**34**:368-376

[42] Hoffer KJ. The Hoffer Q formula: A comparison of theoretic and regression formulas. Journal of Cataract and Refractive Surgery. 1993;**19**:700-712

[43] Holladay JT et al. A three-part system for refining intraocular lens power calculations. Journal of Cataract and Refractive Surgery. 1988;**14**:17-24

[44] Retzlaff JA, Sanders DR, Kraff MC. Development of the SRK/T intraocular lens implant power calculation formula. Journal of Cataract and Refractive Surgery. 1990;**16**:333-340

[45] Goto S et al. Prediction of postoperative intraocular lens position with angle-to-angle depth using anterior segment optical coherence tomography. Ophthalmology. 2016;**123**:2474-2480

[46] Martinez-Enriquez E, Pérez-Merino P, Durán-Poveda S, Jiménez-Alfaro I, Marcos S. Estimation of intraocular lens position from full crystalline lens geometry: Towards a new generation of intraocular lens power calculation formulas. Scientific Reports. 2018;**8**:9829. DOI: 10.1038/s41598-018-28272-6

[47] Satou T, Shimizu K, Tsunehiro S, et al. Development of a new intraocular lens power calculation method based on lens position estimated with optical coherence tomography. Scientific Reports. 2020;**10**:6501. DOI: 10.1038/s41598-020-63546-y

[48] Huang D, Tang M, Wang L, Zhang X, Armour RL, Gattey DM, et al. Optical coherence tomography-based corneal power measurement and intraocular lens power calculation following laser vision correction (an American ophthalmological society thesis). Transactions of the American Ophthalmological Society. 2013;**111**:34-45

[49] Savini G, Hoffer KJ, Balducci N. Comparison of formula accuracy for intraocular lens power calculation based on measurements by a swept-source optical coherence tomography optical biometer. Journal of Cataract and Refractive Surgery. 2020;**46**(1):27-33. DOI: 10.1016/j.jcrs.2019.08.044

[50] Leung EH, Gibbons A, Koch DD. Cost-effectiveness of preoperative OCT in cataract evaluation for multifocal intraocular lens. Ophthalmology. 2020;**127**(7):859-865. DOI: 10.1016/j.ophtha.2020.01.049. Epub 2020 Jan 31